Death, Dying and Palliative Care in Children and Young People

Death, Dying and Palliative Care in Children and Young People: Perspectives from Health Psychology examines the issues relevant to children and young people living with serious illness and their families by taking a closer look at the literature and knowledge around the processes of care, health, well-being and development through a health psychology lens.

The text introduces readers to the general palliative and holistic care needs of children and young people along with the nuances of caring relationships. The chapters discuss the vulnerabilities encountered in living with serious illness and facing a shortened life prognosis, being at the end of life and issues relative to the historical concept of the 'good death' or 'dying well', grief, and bereavement. The author examines how individual and familial experiences can be multi-layered, which can consequently influence perceptions and behaviours. The text therefore offers a deep exploration of the varied ways in which people draw on different resources to navigate their palliative care lived experiences.

The book will be beneficial to the students of, and individuals interested in, psychology and nursing along with other health and social care courses. It will further be of interest to individuals interested in gaining more understanding of the experiential aspects of death, dying and palliative care in children and young people from health psychology perspectives.

Alison M. Rodriguez, PhD, MSc, PCPD, BSc (Hons), is a psychologist with extensive teaching, research and research supervision experience in health and critical health psychology. Alison's current research focuses on the health and well-being of young people with long term, life-limiting and life-threatening conditions.

Death, Dying and Palliative Care in Children and Young People

Perspectives from Health Psychology

Alison M. Rodriguez

Routledge
Taylor & Francis Group
LONDON AND NEW YORK

Designed cover image: © Getty Images

First published 2023
by Routledge
4 Park Square, Milton Park, Abingdon, Oxon OX14 4RN

and by Routledge
605 Third Avenue, New York, NY 10158

Routledge is an imprint of the Taylor & Francis Group, an informa business

British Library Cataloguing-in-Publication Data
A catalogue record for this book is available from the British Library

ISBN: 9781032374406 (hbk)
ISBN: 9781032374420 (pbk)
ISBN: 9781003340287 (ebk)

DOI: 10.4324/9781003340287

Typeset in Bembo
by Newgen Publishing UK

With love to my family
La vida no se trata de esperar a que pase la tormenta ...
se trata de aprender a bailar bajo la lluvia.

Contents

Figures

Tables

About the author

Alison M. Rodriguez PhD, MSc, PCPD, BSc (Hons), is an Associate Professor in Child and Family Health, at the University of Leeds. She is a psychologist (her academic background is health psychology) and Fellow of the Higher Education Academy with extensive teaching, research and research supervision experience in health psychology. Alison's current research focuses on the health and well-being of young people with long term, life-limiting and life-threatening conditions. Her work aims to improve wellbeing, support behaviour change, communication and the quality of care for service users and providers. This involves developing complex psycho-therapeutic and self-management interventions.

See Twitter – ARodriguez339.

https://scholar.google.co.uk/citations?hl=en&hl=en&pli=1&user=NTlRRHAAAAAJ

Preface

Over the last 30 years health psychology has developed as a specialist area of psychology, originally branching away from clinical psychology to focus on the prevention of illness and the maintenance of health and wellbeing; to understand and manage the psychosocial aspects of physical illness. However, it is only in more recent years that health psychology has contributed to the unveiling of the psycho-social demands of death, dying and palliative care for children and young people. Child and family health psychology draws on several overlapping disciplines including developmental psychology.

Palliative care is a generalist and specialist area of healthcare that emanates from the hospice movement and addresses the holistic needs of those with serious illness. A serious illness is *'a health condition that carries a high risk of mortality and either negatively impacts a person's daily function or quality of life, or excessively strains their caregivers'* (Kelley and Bollens-Lund, 2018).

Health psychology provides us with the methodological techniques and theoretical lenses to explore the perceptions and behaviours of individuals, families and professionals toward death and dying and the psychosocial impact of living whilst in receipt of palliative care with advancing disease. There are health psychology interventions and concepts within the field of children and young people's palliative care, that were originally founded in research on children and young people with chronic or long-term conditions (conditions that with good management will not progress to death). For example, in considering the measurement of pain, the impact of stress, and how to promote adjustment, and resilience when the individual/family are also negotiating key developmental milestones.

It has taken time for health psychology however to appreciate that there can be health and wellbeing within the palliative care context for children and young people. When a child or young person is offered palliative care, they can still be in receipt of active treatments and can still hope to achieve a good quality of life over what remains of their life course.

End of life care is actioned when knowledge of the disease trajectory suggests that the individual may have less than twelve months to live. However, with some conditions and age groups this can be difficult to determine. Indeed, children and young people with certain conditions are now living much longer lives with their advancing illnesses than they did historically both due to improvements in care and medical technological advances. However, at the end of life, it is likely that active treatments may cease, and that any medical or pharmacological intervention will be for symptom management, for example to lessen physical pain, breathlessness, or anxiety. Still, the holistic benefits of palliative care can still be experienced at this time.

The health psychology approach to understanding the needs of children and young people in receipt of palliative care, including end of life care, has been outcome driven, drawing upon process and linear models of state, stress, coping and adjustment and on utilising positivistic methods of inquiry (often by proxy), those synonymous with medicine (Murray, 2015). However, individual's experiences of the realities of their finitude or the shortened life expectancies of young family members may be complex and difficult to measure. This book therefore aims to convey an understanding of what these experiences can involve/be like, rather than be a manual on the health psychological concepts of relevance to children and young people with serious illness or be another introductory textbook to health psychology that details psychological interventions in chronic disease/long term conditions.

Although there is a bias towards UK models of care and practices in resource rich countries, the aim of this book is to provide a nuanced understanding of health psychology perspectives; to consider health perceptions, behaviours and experiences that resonate more with the lived experience of death, dying and palliative care in children and young people. How a child, young person or family member may respond to and cope with a diagnosis of a serious illness or with the psychosocial demands of an advanced disease prognosis will be variable. Age and mental capacity, gender, family dynamics, wider support networks, culture, and access to care and support, each influence individuals in these situations.

Overall, this book should help general readers as well as students on psychology, nursing and other health and social care courses to begin to develop a critical appreciation of the psycho-social issues relevant to wellbeing for children and young people in receipt of palliative care and how cultural conceptions and experiences of death and dying can impact the lives of the children, young people and families who may be in our care.

References

Kelley, A.S. and Bollens-Lund, E., 2018. Identifying the population with serious illness: the 'denominator' challenge. *Journal of Palliative Medicine*, *21*(S2), pp. S–7.

Murray, M. ed., 2015. *Critical Health Psychology*. Macmillan International Higher Education.

Acknowledgements

Thank you to the children and young people I have known with serious illness and to those who have participated in my research studies and their families. The experiences you have shared and the empathy and compassion I have witnessed within your families have helped shape my academic interests. I would also like to thank students past and present who have shown an interest in health psychology perspectives on death, dying and palliative care. Your interest and engagement provided me with the motivation to write this book.

Glossary

Anticipatory grief	A process like the process of mourning but occurs before the actual death.
Attachment theory	An evolutionary theory of parent-child relationships that can influence subsequent development.
Beneficence	An act of kindness towards others including moral obligation.
Bereavement	Experiencing the death or loss of another.
Challenging conversations	An interaction between two or more people characterised by heightened emotion, differing viewpoints and a high level of importance for at least one of the two parties involved.
Chronic disease	A condition that lasts for three months or longer and can get worse over time.
COVID-19	A Coronavirus.
Existentialist philosophy	A type of philosophical enquiry that investigated human existence and the subjective experience of thinking, feeling and acting.
Foucauldian	An issue or argument relating to the ideas of the French philosopher Michel Foucault.
Dying well	End of life care that assists individuals with advanced illness to live as well as possible until the point of death.
Good death	An historical concept that suggests a freedom from suffering and a death that is congruent with the individual and families wishes.
Health and social care professionals	People in health and social care roles.
Humanitarian	Human welfare.
Intervention	An action or activity or process of intervening.

Long term condition	An illness that cannot be cured but can be controlled with pharmaceutical intervention.
Mourning	The expression of sorrow.
Non-Western	Areas of the world not including countries of Western Europe and North America.
Normative	Relevant or relating to a standard or behavioural norm.
Palliative care professionals	People in palliative care roles.
Paradigm	An example, perspective or set of ideas.
Pathologised	Regarded or treated as psychologically abnormal.
Resource rich countries	A country that derives at least 20% of exports from non-renewable natural resources.
Resource poor countries	Countries that are poor and low in natural resources.
The West	The western world Europe, North America and Oceania.
The East	The eastern world Central Asia, East Asia, the Greater Middle East, South Asia and Southeast Asia.
Western	Living in or originating from the west.
World Health Organisation	A specialised agency of the United Nations responsible for international public health.

Prologue

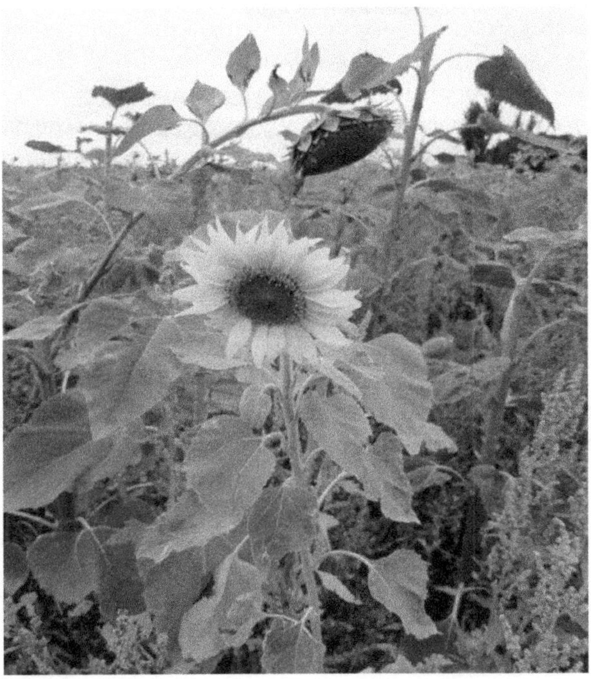

Prologue Figure 1 A photograph of a sunflower in a field of plants. Photograph taken by Alison Rodriguez.

Introduction

The area of healthcare that we identify as 'palliative care' has stemmed from the hospice movement, involving specialist and generalist health and social care services, and is an integral part of the care delivered by health and social care professionals to those living with and dying from a serious illness – any

DOI: 10.4324/9781003340287-1

advanced, progressive, or incurable disease. Palliative care is not just about care in the last months, days, or hours of a person's life (end of life care); it is also about enabling someone to live with a serious illness. This chapter introduces the reader to the need for palliative care for children and young people with serious illness, highlighting current and future projections of disease burden in the UK and globally. Relevant terminology and the various definitions, conceptions and models of palliative care available and across service sectors will be briefly described. There will also be a brief introduction to the barriers that exist for individuals' acceptance of palliative care and related issues of coping. The chapter will then provide an overview of subsequent chapters.

Palliative care need

Palliative care is a global issue; fifty-six million people die annually worldwide. In the UK, it is estimated that by 2040, annual deaths will increase to 628,659. From within this population, it is considered that those who will benefit from palliative care will increase to 469,305 people/year. Certain disease related projections have also been observed, identifying that dementia could increase to 219,409 deaths/year by 2040 and cancer to 208,636 deaths: the two most prevalent disease categories. Countries that have similar population demographic profiles could also observe these future trends (Etkind et al., 2017). (In Chapter 2 there is more focused discussion on the numbers of children and young people currently in receipt of palliative care services).

Sleeman et al. (2019) have published a global projection of the population that will be living with serious illness up to 2060. They used a calculation that included methods adopted by the Lancet commission on palliative care and pain relief assessing global need. They also combined these methods with the World Health Organisation (WHO) global and regional projections of mortality. They suggest that in 2060 we will be seeing that approximately 47% deaths globally will follow serious health related suffering, with 83% of these deaths being within low- and middle-income countries. These figures highlight that 130,000 people worldwide by 2060 will be dying from a serious illness each day. The burden on healthcare, however, is much greater because the calculation is based on deaths and not with consideration of those living with serious illness. The increase in the burden of serious health-related suffering forecasted between 2016 and 2060 will occur in all World Health Organisation (WHO) regions. The regions that will observe the greatest upward trends however will be the eastern Mediterranean (170% increase) and Africa (126% increase), with the largest increase to be observed in the western Pacific region (over six million more people in 2060, 87% increase on figures in 2016). These areas are currently the areas with the least developed palliative care provision integrated into their health care systems.

The 2014 World Health Assembly Resolution 67.19 on *'Strengthening of palliative care as a component of comprehensive care throughout the life course'* (2016) suggested that where there is a need for palliative care, its provision can markedly improve the lives of individuals.

Palliative care, as a person-centred approach to care is also included in the definition of universal health coverage. The WHO global strategy on people-centred and integrated health services (2015) also offers a framework for developing palliative care across disease types globally. More recently, Lucy Watts MBE, a youth ambassador and advocate for children and young people with life limiting conditions had her voice heard at the 2018 WHO assembly, arguing that access to children's palliative care and in particular access to pain relief should also be offered at a global level. In February 2018, Lucy then met with Dr Tedros, the Director General of the WHO, who has since pledged to continue working with Lucy to enable the palliative care needs of children and young people to be met across the world (Jabbarian, 2018).

Palliative care for children and young people, in some contexts referred to paediatric palliative care, is multidisciplinary, supporting children and young people with serious illness and their families from the point of diagnosis and over the duration of their illness trajectory. The provision that is offered is different to adult palliative care because the decision making, symptom management and communication need to be tailored to the child or young person's age or developmental status and be considerate of much greater familial involvement. Children are dependent on parents/guardians and by law their involvement needs be present in treatment and care decision-making (World Health Organisation, 2018).

Definitions and models of palliative care

Palliative care takes different shapes in different regions of the world. Looking at provision broadly both in the UK and overseas, palliative care is delivered in community, hospital and hospice settings. The InsupC project conducted under the European Union 7th Framework Programme investigated longitudinally the best ways to deliver integrated (professionals from multiple services working together) care to individuals with cancer, heart failure or lung disease. The provision of good palliative care is argued to be individual needs focused and flexible enough so that it can be delivered in a place of the individuals and families choosing (Hasselaar and Payne, 2016).

Palliative care is delivered for all age groups with serious illness or advancing disease; for individuals often categorised as living with a life threatening or life limiting condition. Life-limiting (or life-shortening) conditions (TfSL, 2023) are those for which there is no reasonable hope of cure and from which the individual will die, for example:

- Cancer
- Heart disease
- Chronic obstructive pulmonary disease

- Dementia
- Heart failure
- Neuromuscular disease
- Neurodegenerative disease
- Chronic liver disease
- Renal disease.

Life-threatening conditions (TfSL, 2023) are those for which curative treatment may be feasible but can fail. These include:

- Advanced progressive incurable disease
- Where death is expected soon
- When there is a risk of death from an acute crisis in condition
- Where sudden catastrophic events have produced a life-threatening situation
- When the prospect of survival is small, for example extremely premature infants.

The provision of palliative care across the lifespan includes services for individuals with conditions considered life limiting or life threatening. For the purpose of this book, reference will be made to 'serious illness' and relatedly 'advancing disease'. In doing so, these terms are considered all encompassing of the range of conditions that require palliative care and can lead to end of life care and a shortened life prognosis. Historically, a shortened life prognosis would have been discussed using only the word 'terminal'. There is dislike for this word amongst some professionals, academics and individuals who are facing the prospect of the end of their life. Pamela van der Riet (2006), a nurse, highlights some of the reasons for this dislike in reflecting on some of those she has supported through her palliative care practice:

> *'We were told our patient Clara had cancer of the cervix and was admitted for terminal care. How I hate that word 'terminal' as it trivialises dying. Several years ago, a young cancer patient I was interviewing for my doctoral studies had just been told by his doctor that his cancer condition was 'terminal' and he pointed out that the word 'terminal' reminded him of being in a bus station. He said that he was not at a bus station; he was 'dying'!'*
>
> (p, 81)

Moving on to what is meant by palliative care, it is recognised that numerous definitions exist. Palliative care is defined by the World Health Organisation (WHO, 2023) as:

> *An approach that improves the quality of life of patients and their families facing the problems associated with life-threatening illness, through the prevention and relief of suffering by means of early identification and impeccable assessment and treatment of pain and other problems, physical, psychosocial and spiritual.*

Historically, palliative care for adults was provided only when any curative treatment had failed. In more recent years, there has been a drive to offer adults palliative care alongside active treatment and much earlier in disease trajectories. But this can be dependent on the nature and timeline of the condition. In contrast, the child model of care:

> *Begins when illness is diagnosed and continues regardless of whether or not a child receives treatment directed at the disease.*
>
> (WHO, 2023)

Palliative care for children and young people, unlike for adults, may commonly span many months, or years and is family centred. The WHO definition of palliative care for children is therefore separate and is summarised as:

> *'The active total care of the child's body, mind and spirit, and involves giving support to the family'.*
>
> (WHO, 2023)

A working definition for neonatal palliative care, an emerging specialism, is provided by the UK charity Together for Short Lives (TfSL):

> *'Palliative care for a foetus, neonate, or infant with a life limiting condition is an active and total approach to care, from the point of diagnosis or recognition, throughout the child's life, at the time of death and beyond. It embraces physical, emotional, social, and spiritual elements and focuses on the enhancement of quality of life for the neonatal infant and support for the family. It includes the management of distressing symptoms, the provision of short breaks, and care through death and bereavement'.*
>
> (TfSL, 2023)

Where neonatal palliative care may be offered it is usually because of the following three reasons:

1. The infant is born at the threshold of viability, or they are of a similar grade of vulnerability due to being born prematurely.
2. The infant has been born with anomalies that could influence viral functions.
3. The infant is in receipt of intensive care but no longer coping very well with interventions, to a degree where the interventions are no longer beneficial and are being maintained just to prolong life.

It is also now possible to offer palliative care support to parents before a child is born, in situations where there is knowledge about how there are likely to be problems with viability and extending life at birth (Wool, 2013).

Further notes on terminology

Palliative care alongside its different models of service delivery also uses a wealth of additional and diverse terminology:

1. End of Life Care – This aspect of palliative care is focused on the end stage of life, for those categorised with advanced disease. Care is supportive and aimed at meeting the needs of individuals and families into bereavement. Much emphasis is on the management of pain, psycho-social and instrumental support.
2. General(ist) Palliative Care Service – This is palliative care which is delivered in all sectors of health care by providers who also offer care to nonpalliative individuals in their service provision. This care is provided at any time following a life threatening/limiting diagnosis (sometimes prior to diagnosis if the condition is rare yet symptoms are complex and presumed life limiting) and supports the alleviation of symptoms and provides psycho-social support. There is no expectation that cares provided will cure the disease.
3. Hospice care – This is a philosophy of care and so can be provided either in the community or in a hospice-built setting. The hospice care philosophy is focused on improving the lives of people who have a life-limiting or advanced life-threatening illness, helping them to live well and make the most of their lives before they die. Hospice care supports the physical, psycho-social and spiritual needs of individuals. Hospice also has tailored support for the significant others of individuals and their lay carers throughout the individual's advancing disease and their bereavement.
4. Specialist palliative care – This type of palliative care is argued to be the active, total care of individuals with life limiting/threatening conditions. Individuals and families are supported by a multi-professional team, where each member will have completed recognised specialist palliative care training to provide disease relevant physical, psycho-social and spiritual support.
5. Integrated palliative care – Integrated palliative care is a team-based approach that connects relevant expertise and aims to support the physical, psychosocial and spiritual needs of individuals, through identifying the social system of the individual. Integrated palliative care is implemented early in the disease trajectory alongside active or curative interventions. This approach hopes to alleviate individual's suffering through key transitions in their illness and to support place of care choices. Integrative palliative care, however, is still in its infancy in terms of the evidence base. We need to explore how this type of palliative care works with the different health care systems of different countries and how individuals and families experience it.

Therefore, whether one is receiving palliative care at home, in the community, hospital or hospice setting there can also be reference made to end of life care, generalist or specialist palliative care and more recently integrative palliative care (Hasselaar and Payne, 2016).

Barriers to palliative care

The overarching focus of palliative care for all age groups is not on death and dying, it is on living and achieving a quality of life. This focus increasingly supports engaging other services for early referrals to palliative care for those still undergoing active treatment for cure. However, this advanced thinking is not yet adopted by all service models or countries. Stigma or poor understanding of what palliative care is often means that individuals are frightened by the mere mention of palliative or hospice care. Unfortunately, these perceptions can hinder quality of life and lead to more anxiety for individuals and families (Shen and Wellman, 2019).

Furthermore, because health and social care professionals are motivated to maintain hope in the individuals in their care, they can find it difficult to convey to individuals that there is no longer the possibility of cure. Allied to this situation, discussions about preferred place of death and care choices need to be had, which again professionals can be hesitant to talk about. This can lead to individuals and families being unsure about their options. In addition, professionals may lack experience in providing emotional support or the physical symptoms that can accompany the end of life, and so they feel restricted in what advice to give and what options to suggest. Health care professionals are trained to draw on all efforts to prolong life, and therefore can feel like they have given up on an individual if they arrive at a point whereby hopes are dashed and only comfort care can be offered.

It can be easier if individuals and families are prepared for these challenging times and related conversations. In such circumstances they may then feel that they can better express their wishes and without prior direction. They can feel confident to begin discussions, rather than waiting for a critical incident or health crisis that then necessitates quick decisions. Of course, there can be other barriers that stop individuals from voicing their wishes, including their protectiveness of families and in some cases their lack of psychological support that renders their mood to be low and their outlook to be hopeless. In these instances, an individual's motivation to action their choices can be lacking. Unfortunately, mental, and behavioural health care can sometimes be overlooked as an important part of both palliative and end-of-life care in the immediate priority of offering physical comfort and symptom control (Kylmä et al., 2009; Shen and Wellman, 2019). Chapters 4 and 6 further address the vulnerabilities of a shortened life prognosis and issues relative to open communication and advance care planning, and Chapter 7 addresses dying well and the 'good death' for children and young people which has its conceptual and historical roots in resource rich countries where it is understood that adults have an adequate death if they have an awareness of their impending death and have had the opportunity to plan for their eventuality.

Palliative services are growing, thanks to increasing awareness of the benefits of palliative care earlier in disease trajectories and an increasing legitimisation of the approach and philosophy of palliative care across health systems. However, there is still much reliance on families to provide care and to draw on their own resources to be able to cope with the psychosocial, spiritual, and emotional burdens that can be felt from the sense of isolation that can occur whilst supporting a child or young person with palliative care needs at home or in the community. The social aspects of death, dying and palliative care are being highlighted by a new public health palliative care movement (Abel and Kellehear, 2022).

The public health approach to palliative and end of life care

Supporting individuals across the lifespan through their disease and end of life trajectories is something families have always encountered. In resource rich countries we have the access to professional services for guidance and support but in resource poor countries the experience is still very much embedded in communities, with support and guidance from social networks rather than formalised services, or where there is a palliative care service, this may look quite different to the interdisciplinary team approach we see in the UK and other resource rich countries. Although we may argue that there is much need in these resource poor communities to fund better pain and other medical interventions to ease suffering, it is possible that the community cohesion that has been maintained in these societies is something that we in resource rich countries can relearn.

The public health approach to palliative care (Abel and Kellehear, 2016) aims to harness community 'assets and capacity' to better enable those who want to support family members with serious disease. It is commonplace for example for individuals to politely refuse offers of help from their community, but this approach argues that for our culture to change, then we must begin to accept help from others in our community and to accept help early on in disease trajectories. This will mean that later the support is already there, and families are then not left to be alone struggling emotionally or fighting in small family units, unable to access resources due to service criteria or capacity. With community help, families then may have more time and mental space to manage everything.

As stated by Abel and Kellehear, 2022 (p768):

> *It is the social context of dying that provides the basis for public health palliative care. This is not a rejection of symptom science as an important dimension of the practice of palliative medicine. Rather, this is an expansion of existing practice models to include not just the person with the illness, but also the networks of care that surround them. It includes the supportive relationships between the members of networks. Health and well-being is intimately linked to social ecology.*

The movement has started by creating compassionate policies and with this ethos, recognising compassionate cities. For example, if local councils develop policy guidance for schools, colleges, and workplaces to socially support individuals with serious illness and their families, then they can become more involved with individuals and families in need. The approach recognises that volunteering is a valuable resource; communities have the capacity to support each other and without the need to be bound together as a formal service initiative. We are in the early years of this movement, but it is building pace and motivating professionals from a wide range of disciplinary backgrounds to become more death, dying and palliative care aware and aware of the influence of people's social histories and current social circumstances on their more holistic health and wellbeing statuses. Throughout this book we acknowledge social factors as they also resonate with taking a health psychology perspective toward death, dying and palliative care in children and young people.

Coping

To deal with major stressors in our lives we employ ways or strategies to manage the demands or burdens we feel; this is otherwise conceptualised as coping (Lazarus and Folkman, 1984). At the point of serious illness diagnosis and for many also the time waiting and leading up to the 'news', can engage individuals and their families in a whirlwind of emotions relating to worrying about the everyday practical implications of ill health to concerns about the social, psychological, and existential impacts of the condition. To adjust to life with a given diagnosis and prognosis (understanding what may be ahead in terms of the illness, complexity, care, and timeline) we need to enact various coping strategies, which can also change over time to manage and adjust and to try and maintain wellbeing (Folkman and Lazarus, 1988).

To enable academics to study coping and adjustment within health contexts, coping efforts have been categorised into three main types of strategies:

- Problem-focused – where the strategy focus is on the root cause of the stressor, changing one's attitudes or behaviours toward it.
- Emotion-focused – where there are cognitive efforts enacted to reduce the perceived stress from the stressor.
- Meaning-focused – where regardless of the stress, efforts are focused on maintaining positivity and wellbeing for themselves and others (Folkman and Greer, 2000).

The literature also identifies strategies that involve engagement or disengagement with the stressor. Those with serious illness or those caring for a child or young person with serious illness may find both engagement and disengagement works for them; at times they may need to withdraw from the stressor or avoid it and at other times they may need to deal with it directly. How and when can be determined by the person's psychological wellbeing, emotions, and social situation.

Liao et al. (2018) chartered the stressors and coping foci of individuals throughout their disease trajectories, from diagnosis to being at the close of their lives. Initial stressors included physical symptoms, loss of physical functioning, persistent uncertainty and how to manage their condition. Individuals will draw on previously adopted strategies, ones that have helped them with stressors in the past. However, over time, as individuals adjust to living with their serious illness their coping develops to involve an array of strategies including finding ways to stay positive, trying not to mull over their illness, actively searching for social support, trying to keep up with everyday activities to maintain a sense of normality, modifying expectations, reaching degrees of acceptance of their life situation, and seeking out religious and spiritual ways of coping (Walshe et al., 2017). Individuals can also find that they can grow emotionally through this experience and find a deeper sense of meaning for their lives lived and their purpose in life (Chochinov, 2012).

Coping with advancing disease and living with serious illness can be an experience that has high and low peaks in emotions. Individuals can live one day feeling that they can cope with what is happening to them and the next day they may struggle. Where there is death awareness, emotions may oscillate between feeling that they can face death and dying to not being able to think about their end of life at all. Somewhere on this continuum of thoughts are the days where they will feel more optimistic about their time left and how they can still create memories and have meaningful moments in their life (Sand et al., 2009, 2018).

Receiving a serious illness diagnosis does move one's thoughts then to prognosis. Health and social care professionals when discussing prognosis with individuals and families, will try to encourage effective coping strategies. These include the promotion of the individual's control over their symptoms, to helping families to identify and support symptom management, offering practical and emotional support, goal setting, encouraging them to live in the moment and the needs of today and by doing so, helping them to try and balance the need to retain some level of hope for living alongside the reality of the prognosis.

Palliative care supporting coping

As noted, on diagnosis and in the days and weeks that follow, people will aim to draw on their previously used and successful coping strategies. Palliative care professionals will try to determine what these coping strategies are and support individuals to see that these same strategies can work for them here too – it is important that individuals try their best to draw on the resources they have than to immediately slump into a situation of feeling they have no control. Unsurprisingly individuals/families can feel a great loss of self on diagnosis/prognosis and feel unable to draw on their previous ways of being at such an upsetting time or because of their functionality due to disease progression or the effects of treatment. Professionals will support individuals and families to process their loss and the grief they are feeling whilst at the same time introduce to them effective ways of coping (see Table prologue 1) (Greer et al., 2018, 2020; Jacobsen et al., 2014).

Prologue Table 1 Effective ways of coping

Coping Category	*Strategy*	*Examples*
Cognitive	Self-distraction	Doing something creative, working, engaging in physical activity.
	Cognitive restructuring	Identifying and delineating or making sense out of negative thoughts.
	Mindfulness	Focusing on the here and now, engaging in meditation or yoga exercise.
Behavioural	Problem solving	Identify problems, set goals, put together an action plan.
	Accessing social support	Identify ways you can access support from others to meet your practical and emotional needs.
	Behavioural activation	Think about your values and how you can maintain them. Keep doing day to day what you enjoy doing for as long as you can.
Emotional and physical	Physical interventions	Pace yourself but engage in physical activity, try to sleep well, learn, and engage in relaxation exercises.
	Positive psychology	Think about how you can look forward to positive activities in the future. Hope for pleasant things to happen for yourself and others. Tell others you care/love/appreciate them. Laugh and laugh with others.
	Flow	Hobbies, creativity, work.
Existential (Spiritual)	Religion/spirituality	Pray, visit services at places of worship.
	Life review	Write letters to our loved ones. Consider a 'bucket' list, Begin a legacy project. Reconcile with loved ones.
	Meaning making	Think about your personal growth, the positive things that have happened and how you can still achieve new goals.
	Acceptance	Be 'real' with others. Share with loved ones what goals you would like to achieve.

Source: Adapted from Jacobsen et al., 2014 as cited in Greer et al., 2020.

Moving palliative care to the outpatient setting and earlier in the disease trajectory has meant that professionals outside of specialist palliative care provision have needed to develop new skills. These skills are supported by training in how to assess, support, and teach effective coping strategies (Hui and Bruera, 2016).

Health psychology perspectives

Health psychology has a place and purpose in several key areas of children and young person's palliative care provision (Thompson and Kentor, 2021).

Assessment – Health psychology assists health and social care professionals to determine the differences between coping and maladjustment and to know when individuals are struggling with their mental health. This is promoted using comprehensive interviewing techniques, and by using standardised and validated tools to screen and measure coping and psychological outcomes. Any judgement of normative or maladaptive coping is also influenced by knowledge of normative child development. Health psychology knowledge also supports health and social care professionals to assess cognitive function and decision-making ability, and any complicated grief reaction.

Intervention – Health psychology has influenced interventions to support adjustment to illness, treatment, hospitalisation, side effects, health status changes and bodily limitations. Evidence based interventions have been developed to address emotional and behavioural symptoms, for example they have encouraged the use of cognitive behaviour therapy techniques for some children and young people to enable their coping. Interventions that promote nonpharmacological pain and symptom management have also been developed, for example distraction, mindfulness and relaxation techniques have been promoted to help with fatigue, sleep problems and nausea. Health psychology approaches to communication delivery can also support individuals and families in decision-making and advocate the child or young persons voice in their treatment plans. Health psychology research has highlighted the emotional support needs of children, young people, care givers and siblings and has advocated the need for meaning making and early bereavement support.

Consultation – Health psychology has facilitated communication between families and health and social care professionals and communication within multidisciplinary teams. Health psychology studies have involved much collaboration with different professional groups to aide the development of tools to guide conversations with individuals and families and to successfully evaluate outcomes.

Chapter summary and book overview

In this short prologue, current conceptualisations of palliative care and practice are introduced. Added to this it is highlighted how stress and coping are issues faced by those with serious and advancing illness and it is discussed how palliative care has a role to play in both alleviating stress and in assisting with enhancing coping efforts for children, young people and families. Living with a serious illness involves periods of adjustment and efforts to maintain one's quality of life and a positive outlook.

In Chapter 1 the history of palliative care is provided, detailing the hospice movement and a summary overview of the key thinkers that have influenced contemporary views toward spirituality and existentialism, each influencing our perceptions and behaviours toward death and dying and in living with and supporting children and young people with serious and advancing illness and their families.

In Chapter 2 a lifespan approach to understanding the perceptions, behaviours, and experiences of children and young people in receipt of palliative care or living with death and dying is offered. The lifespan perspective within health psychology influences how we consider supporting individuals with serious illness and their families considering their age and developmental stage. We can appreciate that at different life stages there are different developmental needs and changes that are also situated in diverse socio-cultural contexts.

In Chapter 3, caring relationships within palliative care are considered, assisted by discussion of the constructs of empathy, compassion, and mutuality. Their implications for palliative care and person and family centredness are explored. At the centre of palliative 'care' are the 'care' relationships, which are the relational experiences. Whether we can teach compassion will be considered. Self-care and emotional distancing are also discussed as relevant to palliative care practice and the changing nature of our worlds, especially considering social media usage amongst individuals and families. The chapter highlights the complexity of relationships within the context palliative care.

In Chapter 4, the perceived vulnerabilities that accompany a shortened life prognosis for children and young people will be considered, introducing the reader to the impacts of shortened life awareness and the concept of truth telling in the context of palliative care. The chapter highlights the need to be diverse in palliative care practices to accommodate the needs of individuals and families. The notion of the 'patient as vulnerable' holds prominence with respect to age, condition, and diverse cultural and ethical belief systems. These nuances are explored, and issues around bad news delivery, concealment and mutual pretense highlighted.

In Chapter 5, the paradox of living whilst dying is further explored and the extent to which meaning making through reflecting on memories, life storying and legacy leaving supports wellbeing is considered. It will be highlighted how health and social care professionals can validate individual's existential explorations through an unfolding life storying dialogue. Individuals can find meaning and a continued reason for life (Sartre's notion of 'raison d'etre') by professionals supporting them to reflect on their past, find peace with their present, and cognitively and emotionally manage their futures. This can also be both a rewarding and challenging task for professionals.

In Chapter 6, the lived experience of serious illness and advancing disease is considered in depth, by exploring the liminality and embodiment of illness, the experience of suffering and 'total pain'. The biographical disruption that palliative care both contributes to, and supports is considered against the instrumental support that can be provided to individuals and families to enable them to attach a 'silver lining' to their lived experiences. In this chapter we also consider palliative care in situations of crisis, discussing how and in what ways humanitarian crises of war and pandemics can impact on experiences.

In Chapter 7, we consider the historical concept of a 'good' or 'good enough' death and consider its contemporary relevance to 'dying well'. The definitional challenges of determining the biomedical bodily death will be highlighted and the diverse cultural and religious persuasions of being towards the 'good' death will be explored. Palliative care supports individuals on their 'journey' of living with serious illness and advancing disease and of course in dying. To enhance care, professionals can embrace cultural expectations and offer a combined person and family centred approach to palliative care. It is of importance to individuals and families that their existential and spiritual belief systems are acknowledged and in doing so, they can also feel supported psycho-socially. Here there is a spotlight placed upon autonomy and dignity in palliative care. We consider ways professionals can support children, young people and families to meet their palliative and end of life wishes. Different patient groups have different trajectories towards their deaths, yet most experience some degree of death anxiety. This can have implications for the 'good' death or 'dying well' and how palliative care is shaped and received. The challenges posed to achieve a 'good death' and a supportive palliative care experience for children and young people with palliative care needs will be exemplified.

Children and young people's palliative care came about much later than adult palliative care and as the specialism develops we are increasingly aware of the support needs of families. It is important that we are mindful of the unique needs of children and young people and other developmentally delayed groups as understandings of their predicaments can be linked to their developmental status. This area of care for children and young people is still in its infancy with much more research to do and things to learn to benefit children and young people and their families.

Following discussion around 'good' death frameworks, the needs of families in the care of the deceased are highlighted. Funerals further highlight the needs of mourners to involve themselves in ritual, out of respect for the deceased and to accommodate their spiritual belief systems.

In Chapter 8, historical and theoretical conceptions of grief are explored. Following, the degree to which new theoretical understandings of grief have brought about change in palliative care practice and bereavement support is debated. Bereavement can occur at any age and involve different relationships and psycho-social demands. The implications of several types of bereavement will be explored and further how our different experiences can affect how grief and bereavement can be internalised, externalised, and managed differently in different communities and within children and young people's palliative care.

In the epilogue the main contributions of the book are reflected upon. Considering what can be learnt and taken away for professionals to consider in their practice, for scholars to further muse over theoretically and critically and for researchers to empirically study further.

References

Abel, J. and Kellehear, A., 2016. Palliative care reimagined: a needed shift. *BMJ Supportive & Palliative Care*, *6*(1), pp.21–26.

Abel, J. and Kellehear, A., 2022. Public health palliative care: Reframing death, dying, loss and caregiving. *Palliative Medicine*, *36*(5), pp.768–769.

Chochinov, H.M., 2012. *Dignity therapy: Final words for final days*. OUP USA.

Etkind, S.N., Bone, A.E., Gomes, B., Lovell, N., Evans, C.J., Higginson, I.J. and Murtagh, F.E.M., 2017. How many people will need palliative care in 2040? Past trends, future projections, and implications for services. *BMC Medicine*, *15*(1), pp.1–10.

Folkman, S. and Greer, S., 2000. Promoting psychological well-being in the face of serious illness: when theory, research and practice inform each other. *Psycho-Oncology: Journal of the Psychological, Social and Behavioural Dimensions of Cancer*, *9*(1), pp.11–19.

Folkman, S., and Lazarus, R.S., 1988. Coping as a mediator of emotion. *Journal of Personality and Social Psychology*, *54*(3), p.466.

Greer, J.A., Applebaum, A.J., Jacobsen, J.C., Temel, J.S. and Jackson, V.A., 2020. Understanding and addressing the role of coping in palliative care for patients with advanced cancer. *Journal of Clinical Oncology*, *38*(9), p.915.

Greer, J.A., Jacobs, J.M., El-Jawahri, A., Nipp, R.D., Gallagher, E.R., Pirl, W.F., Park, E.R., Muzikansky, A., Jacobsen, J.C., Jackson, V.A. and Temel, J.S., 2018. Role of patient coping strategies in understanding the effects of early palliative care on quality of life and mood. *Journal of Clinical Oncology*, *36*(1), p.53.

Hasselaar, J. and Payne, S., 2016. *Integrated palliative care*. Nijmegan: Radboud University Medical Centre.

Hui, D. and Bruera, E., 2016. Integrating palliative care into the trajectory of cancer care. *Nature reviews Clinical Oncology*, *13*(3), pp.159–171.

Jabbarian, L., 2018. Lucy Watts meets Dr Tedros. EAPC Blog.

Jacobsen, J., Kvale, E., Rabow, M., Rinaldi, S., Cohen, S., Weissman, D. and Jackson, V., 2014. Helping patients with serious illness live well through the promotion of adaptive coping: a report from the improving outpatient palliative care (IPAL-OP) initiative. *Journal of Palliative Medicine*, *17*(4), pp.463–468.

Kylmä, J., Duggleby, W., Cooper, D. and Molander, G., 2009. Hope in palliative care: an integrative review. *Palliative & Supportive Care*, 7(3), pp.365–377.

Lazarus, R.S. and Folkman, S., 1984. *Stress, appraisal, and coping*. Springer Publishing Company.

Liao, Y.C., Liao, W.Y., Sun, J.L., Ko, J.C. and Yu, C.J., 2018. Psychological distress and coping strategies among women with incurable lung cancer: a qualitative study. *Supportive Care in Cancer*, *26*(3), pp.989–996.

Riet, P.V.D., 2006. A palliative care story: Negotiating the abject. *Contemporary Nurse*, *22*(1), pp.81–83.

Sand, L., Olsson, M. and Strang, P., 2009. Coping strategies in the presence of one's own impending death from cancer. *Journal of Pain and Symptom Management*, *37*(1), pp.13–22.

Sand, L., Olsson, M. and Strang, P., 2018. Supporting in an existential crisis: A mixed-methods evaluation of a training model in palliative care. *Palliative & Supportive Care*, *16*(4), pp.470–478.

Shen, M.J. and Wellman, J.D., 2019. Evidence of palliative care stigma: The role of negative stereotypes in preventing willingness to use palliative care. *Palliative & Supportive Care*, *17*(4), pp.374–380.

Sleeman, K.E., De Brito, M., Etkind, S., Nkhoma, K., Guo, P., Higginson, I.J., Gomes, B. and Harding, R., 2019. The escalating global burden of serious health-related suffering: projections to 2060 by world regions, age groups, and health conditions. *The Lancet Global Health*, 7(7), pp. e883–e892.

Thompson, A.L., and Kentor, R.A., 2021. Introduction to the special issue on palliative, end of life, and bereavement: Integrating psychology into paediatric palliative care. *Clinical Practice in Pediatric Psychology*, *9*(3) 219–228.

Together for Short Lives (TfSL) (n.d.) (b) Children's Palliative Care Definitions [Online] Available from: www.togetherforshortlives.org.uk/assets/0000/4089/CPC_definitions.pdf (accessed 3 January 2023).

Walshe, C., Roberts, D., Appleton, L., Calman, L., Large, P., Lloyd-Williams, M. and Grande, G., 2017. Coping well with advanced cancer: a serial qualitative interview study with patients and family carers. *PloS One*, *12*(1), p.e0169071.

Wool, C., 2013. State of the science on perinatal palliative care. *Journal of Obstetric, Gynaecologic & Neonatal Nursing*, *42*(3), pp.372–382.

World Health Organisation Definition of palliative care/WHO Definition of palliative care for children. Geneva: World Health Organization; 2002 www.who.int/cancer/palliative/definition/en/ (accessed 3 January 2023).

World Health Organisation, 2014. Resolution WHA 67/19. Strengthening of palliative care as a component of comprehensive care throughout the life course. Web site. http://apps.who.int/gb/ebwha/pdf_files/ WHA67/A67_R19-en.pdf.

World Health Organisation, 2015. *WHO global strategy on people-centred and integrated health services: interim report* (No. WHO/HIS/SDS/2015.6). World Health Organization.

World Health Organisation, 2018. Technical report: pricing of cancer medicines and its impacts: a comprehensive technical report for the World Health Assembly Resolution 70.12: operative paragraph 2.9 on pricing approaches and their impacts on availability and affordability of medicines for the prevention and treatment of cancer.

1 The underpinnings of children and young people's palliative care

Hospice, spirituality, and existentialism

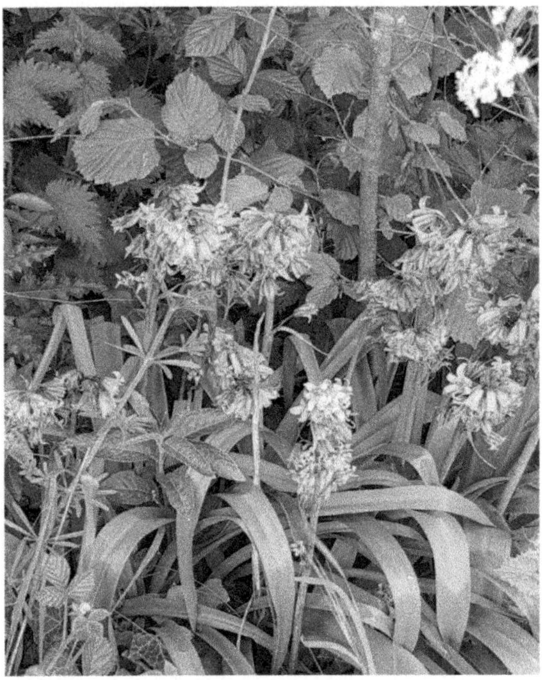

Figure 1.1 Photograph of bluebells, plants, and nettles.
Photograph taken by Alison Rodriguez.

Introduction

The area of health care that we identify as palliative care, stemmed from the hospice movement. The hospice movement was originally summarised as being a *'social movement that augmented and opposed mainstream curative medicine as the hegemonic model of care'* (Syme and Bruce, 2009, p. 20). Analysis of Dame Cicely

DOI: 10.4324/9781003340287-2

Saunders' writings, the founder of the modern hospice movement, suggest that her original intentions, however, were to *'improve and extend medical care at the end of life. The debate of course was around the precise form which this medicine should take'* (Clark and Seymour, 1999, p. 64).

Palliative care in all its guises is built upon the premise of holistic care. A defining feature of palliative care, however, is its attention to spiritual care and spirituality, which is paramount for individuals as they face advancing disease and the end of their lives and for their families as they anticipate their loss (Puchalski et al., 2020). Studies have shown that spiritual wellbeing impacts on the experience of physical symptoms and wellbeing and that psychological symptoms can be heightened if the individual has unresolved spiritual needs or distress (Bultz and Butow, 2011; Salsman et al., 2015). Social roles also change shape through the journey of palliative care and spirituality has been found to impact on these and other relational areas of life (Park et al., 2015; Rego and Nunes, 2019).

Health and social care professionals who work within palliative care are not naïve to individual's experiences of suffering and will at times bear witness to fear, loss, sadness, anger, and guilt. Children, young people and families can emotionally struggle with the physical suffering, burden, loneliness, meaninglessness, and the purpose of their lives. Individuals may indicate freely their need to communicate about these matters, others may require a little encouragement. There is also a current appreciation of how exploring these issues with individuals and their related emotions, relative to their stage of emotional and cognitive development, can be both needed and therapeutic.

Existential psychotherapies or supportive spiritual interventions in palliative care (some of which are discussed further in Chapter 6) are rooted in existential philosophy, otherwise termed existentialism. The key ideas of existential philosophers will be highlighted in this chapter preceded by a summary review of the hospice movement to assist readers in understanding the two intertwined approaches to care. The chapter will highlight the importance of spirituality in providing appropriate palliative care for all that need it.

The hospice movement

The term 'hospice' was taken from its original meaning of 'house of rest and entertainment for pilgrims, travellers or stranger for the destitute or the sick' (Oxford English Dictionary, 2018). The term has been adopted in the sense that a hospice has its doors open to those who are travelling from this life to the next (Craven and Wald, 1975).

In 1902, five of the Sisters of Charity founded St Joseph's Convent in the East End of London and started visiting the sick at home, they also opened St Josephs as a 30-bed establishment for the dying. Following this, St Luke's Hospice was opened in Bayswater, UK. These were two examples of the forerunners of current hospice care, where people were taught the skills needed to support the dying. Two further key historical developments influenced the hospice movement. Firstly, the Marie Curie foundation, which was founded with the purpose to fight the causes of cancer and in their initial review of need, the foundation discusses hospice care. And secondly, the appointment of Dame Cicely Saunders to St Joseph's Hospice in the 1950s as a full time Medical Officer.

The hospice movement was pioneered in England and remains a major source of support and treatment for the populations that can access such care. A key goal of hospice care is to enable people to be comfortable and pain free and to remain as conscious of life as possible, even during the final stages of their lives. Hospices for children and young people are also a source of respite care for families and provide families with specialist advice to assist in their day-to-day cares. The hospice goals are reached via the skills and dedicated philosophies of palliative care, influenced greatly by the foundational work of Dame Cicely Saunders.

Dr Saunders prior to her medical training had also trained as a nurse and social worker. Following her graduation in medicine she researched narcotics and pledged that pain for those dying was not necessary. Still, at this time hospitals were the place to die and practitioners whose focus was on cure, demoted the importance of end-of-life care. However, Saunders (1965) wrote vividly about her exchanges with the dying and how they expressed feelings of guilt, rejection and failure. She saw this as reflective of the attitudes of those held responsible for their cares in the hospital settings and wrote that *'Death is feared, all thoughts of it are avoided, and the dying themselves are often left in loneliness… and are emotionally isolated'* (p70).

Dame Saunders later influenced the opening of St Christopher's hospice; the hospice other adult hospices have since been modelled upon. Her motivations were resultant of her cares for a young Polish man whom she had met on a general surgical ward back in 1948. Although he was physically comfortable in living with his serious illness, he was in extreme emotional pain. Saunders tried to provide emotional comfort to him and engaged in non-medical focused conversations with him. He disclosed his hope that a home could be built for individuals with similar conditions. Days before his death he told Saunders that he was leaving £500 in his 'will' to contribute to this dream (Saunders, 1965).

The following 19 years saw the £500 increase to a sum of £500,000. Saunders had completed her medical training and had gained experience in hospice work, developing her pain reduction techniques. It was then in 1967 that Saunders opened the renowned St Christopher's hospice in Sydenham where there stands proudly, a memorial plaque of the young man who pledged his money for its building.

The USA took longer to embrace the hospice movement. It has been suggested that this was possibly because of the strong cultural persuasion to treat at all costs and that death was often perceived as a weakness. The recognised need for a different approach to the care of the dying was from the scholarship of Elisabeth Kubler-Ross and her work 'On Death and Dying'. Her work was first published in England in 1970 and highlighted the issues of dying in public settings. At the same time, the Vietnam War was in full throw and the American establishment was being critiqued for their treatment of the dying and infirm (Kubler-Ross, 2009).

Palliative Care

Once the Americans acknowledged the potential benefits of hospice care, the hospice movement rapidly gained interest. In Canada, Balfour Mount, then a prominent urologist and cancer surgeon, supported the hospice movement but suggested that the term 'palliative care' be used rather than 'hospice'. This was because 'hospice' posed a language difficulty for the French speakers of Canada. In French, the term 'hospice' means 'alms-house' (a place for the poor) (Henderson et al., 2007). The ethos of palliative care has since been embraced worldwide (Clark et al., 2015).

A large remit of palliative care remains focused on pain control and physical symptom management. However, the palliative care approach or 'philosophy' also recognises the psychosocial demands of conditions and their impact on the social, psychological, and spiritual wellbeing of individuals and their families.

Contemporary hospice provision

Hospices were originally built because there were major gaps in provision for those with advanced cancer conditions. Individuals with cancer remain the largest population of adult hospice care users and still most of the hospice care is funded by charitable sources. In the UK just 32% of hospice care is funded by the NHS (Hospice UK, 2022; Parkinson, 2015). There is, however, building pressure on hospice provision to provide care and support to more people, not least because individuals are living longer with their serious illnesses and because we are seeing the benefits of palliative care when offered earlier in disease trajectories. In 2017, Hospice UK, the national membership body for hospice provision in the UK, launched the initiative 'Open Up Hospice Care', stating '1 in 4 people who need palliative care are not receiving it'.

In 1987 palliative medicine as a medical speciality moved hospice provision into the arena of specialist palliative care. Referrals were then only for those deemed to have medically complex conditions that required the expert care and skills of a team with specialist training. Therefore, hospices have not offered routine care to individuals with serious illness or advancing disease if there was no element of complexity. However, due to population changes and demand, we are seeing hospices are beginning to blur their eligibility criteria to try and care for more people. There is also an active move for adult hospices to be more considerate of individuals needing support who do not have cancer, not least because the *'Commission into the Future of Hospice Care' report highlighted public comments such as 'if you don't have cancer, you're almost treated as a second-class citizen'* (Calanzani et al., 2013, p17).

What about the children?

The first children's hospice was not opened until 1982. Sister Frances Dominica established this hospice following her engagement with a family who turned to her for help when their child Helen was just two years old and was dying from a brain tumour, the year was 1978. Helen had been in hospital for six months and Sister Dominica had got to know the family in that time. At the end of the six months the family were told that there was no longer any hope of recovery. The family knew they wanted to spend the rest of Helens days at home, but Helen needed 24-hour care and there was no detail about how long Helen's remaining life may be. As the time went by Helen's parents were exhausted, receiving no help and feeling increasingly isolated. Sister Dominica, after three months of the family being home, could bear it no longer and offered respite care. They accepted and Sister Dominica would take over the care of Helen from time to time to allow her parents rest, time with their other children or to take a break away from home.

Sister Frances commented in a BBC media article, November (2009):

> *I began to think, if it's helpful to this family, are there other families out there who could benefit?*

This was the beginning of Helen House, the world's first children's hospice.

Sister Frances claimed:

> *The most important people in the planning of Helen House were Helen's parents. From the start we knew it would be small and flexible, it would provide one to one care and the real experts would be the families. The model for the building was home, rather than hospital, the furnishings were things that children would enjoy having in their bedrooms.*

Helen House now also accommodates a unit for young adults aged 18 to 40 years. Together they offer professional care and support to approximately 250 children and young adults, as well as their families. The UK has since seen the development of over forty hospice care facilities for children and young people and provision is growing globally.

When a child is faced with a life limiting/threatening condition it is a social drama as children are the most valued beings of our times. A child dying causes great imbalance and distress in families and the societies to which they belong. Supportive models of care and tailored interventions need to address the developmental stage of the child, their psychosocial and spiritual needs and be ready to accommodate the unpredictability of their physical and emotional responses to therapies, especially regarding the process of dying and the moment of death.

Sister Dominica, then vice president for together for short lives commented in their 2012 'guidance for children's end of life care' document (2012, p5):

> *There can be few greater tragedies for a family than the death of their child. The circumstances surrounding their child's death can have huge impact on family members and can imprint memories which may last a lifetime.*

Spirituality and palliative care

Historically, discussions around spirituality and spiritual care or needs were aligned with a person's religion or faith. Palliative care has broadened our understanding of the spirituality concept:

> *Spirituality is the dynamic dimension of human life that relates to the way persons (individual and community) experience, express and/or seek meaning, purpose and transcendence, and the way they connect to the moment, to self, to others, to nature, to the significant, and/or the sacred.*
>
> (EPICC, 2022)

Dossey (2014) highlights how many consider spirituality and religion with the same sentiment and use the terms interchangeably. However, for those supporting children and young people with serious illness and advancing disease, it is important that they appreciate the differences between the two concepts, not least to support those without a distinct and guiding religious faith. Spiritual care is a means to help individuals to recognise their inner selves and personal life quests. It is a supportive strategy for recognising a person's individuality. In being present, listening and adopting an open stance to this individuality, spiritual care allows the person facing their shortened life trajectory or their family members, to feel they can share their beliefs and values and their emotions. A finite purpose of spiritual care is to support the individual to feel at peace with themselves and the situation they have found themselves in, and to accept that we do not have all the answers and that is OK.

Entwined with providing spiritual care is the need to provide culturally appropriate, or culturally sensitive care. The goal in such is to be or become mindful of an individual's beliefs, values, traditions, and practices and to respect them even if these are diverse, are not in alignment with your own beliefs and values and do not sit with your presumptions about their religion or ethnicity. It is important to not generalise an individual's way of being. For example, not everyone who is catholic goes to church, but their belief in God may still be especially important to them and they may still feel the need to pray, or not.

However, in appreciating these individual differences we still need to consider that our cultural heritage can exert some influence on our beliefs and behaviours. For example, such can influence our expression and meaning of pain and suffering, our attitudes towards bad news disclosure and prognostic awareness, beliefs about the cause and meaning of illness, our readiness for medical interventions and seeking out alterative therapeutic efforts, our attitudes toward death, beliefs about any afterlife, the value of human life and rituals post death for loved ones, and expressions of grief and loss.

In good palliative care provision, spiritual assessment is prioritised alongside the assessment of physical needs. It is with regret to note that in some settings exploring the spiritual needs of individuals and families is not prioritised or limited to detailing the individual's religious choices. This is sometimes because it is presumed that spiritual care is the specialist remit of religious leaders and chaplains and therefore not the responsibility of all other palliative care professionals who should be considerate of individuals' spiritual needs.

Studies conducted to date have been descriptive in nature looking at individual's spiritual needs and not exploring ways of how best those needs can be met (Dos Santos et al., 2022; Hindmarch et al., 2022; Tobi et al., 2022). Individuals struggle most with issues related to their spiritual, existential, and emotional distress. Leading to feelings of hopelessness, frustration and being overwhelmed. Existential and spiritual distress can be of a different duration and nature for everyone, but we are aware of some of the natures of concern. The distress can increase as individuals get closer to death and some individuals experience more existential than physical suffering (Rosa et al., 2022).

Where there has been attention paid to spiritual interventions there is support that many spiritual practices could be guided by all professionals involved in the palliative care of the child or young person and family. Interventions range from the simplest taken for granted compassionate aspects of care such as being present and listening, to actively being involved in the individual's need to leave a legacy, to explore how their life has had meaning and purpose (Rosa et al., 2022). These cares can also help individuals to manage the uncertainty of their disease trajectories and to maintain hope despite their prognosis. Brietbart et al. (2012) developed meaning-focused psychotherapy and Chochinov (2012), Dignity Therapy. Each intervention is aimed to support spiritual need and can be delivered by any trained member of the palliative care team. More discussion of meaning making, and related psychotherapeutic interventions can be found in Chapter 6 and a discussion around what advances in research and practice have been undertaken to amend and develop interventions for children, young people and families.

Spirituality and existentialism

As already noted, a defining feature of palliative care is its attention to spiritual care and spirituality, which is paramount for individuals as they face the end of their lives and for families as they anticipate their loss (Rosa et al., 2022).

The concept of 'Existentialism' has evolved from our notion of 'existence', in that we hold some presence in our life worlds. Heidegger speaks of 'Ek-sistenz', which means 'to stand out from' and suggests we as individuals can stand away from our present being. He states that:

> *The analysis of the characteristics of the being of Da-sein [being there] is an existential one. This means that the characteristics are not properties of something objectively present, but essentially existential ways to be.*
>
> (Heidegger, 1996, p. 126)

We are 'thrown' into culture, language and whether one is male or female. Our 'facticity' or 'thrownness' also influences how we make sense of ourselves and the world in which we inhabit. Heidegger used the term 'existentiell' which he suggests means self-understanding. It is through existence that we develop this self-understanding, *'we come to terms with the question of existence always only through existence itself…existentiell understanding'* (Heidegger, 1996, p. 10). It is the questions of existence that enable us to understand our being, not the metaphysical thinking around what our being may be, but what our meaning and purpose is. It is this thinking that helps us to develop our spirituality. Our spirituality engenders our searching for meaning and purpose in life and our questioning of the meaning of our existence. Our frameworks of thinking around these matters may also be influenced by religious and non-religious belief systems.

We are all culturally and existentially embedded, and so, as we try and make sense of who we are, our identities and the meaning and purpose of our lives, we are doing so from an already existent horizon, driven by the meanings already ascribed by our historicity and culture. We do still however have agency that allows us to develop opinions and choose how to behave. We have a degree of freedom with respect to how we respond to the meanings we derive from the cultures to which we belong. To this end, there is a void between our guiding cultural frameworks and the meanings we ascribe to them which have personal relativity. Chater (2000) suggests that it is this void or middle ground of meaning making that we can conceptualise as our spirituality, stating that it is 'The pain-filled struggle with the contradictions in and between personal life-experience and received, authoritative wisdom. It is a place of contradiction, conflict, pain, and growth' (p. 200). There is understanding that spiritual development involves a struggle of being, to decide what meanings are of most relevance or of importance to one's life lived (Chater, 2020).

Existential theory does not aim to seek answers for life events, but it posits to support individuals in reaching their authentic and most spiritual self as the product of making sense of those events. It is philosophised that throughout our lives we strive to make meaning of our lives, ourselves, and the lives of others. Being told or knowing that we have a shortened life can make our life experiences more meaningful and purposeful. With the end of our lives in sight, it is argued that we become more acutely present of the moment (Montross-Thomas et al., 2018).

The influential thinkers

All existential theorists are united in believing that it is our human pursuit to establish our unique meaning of existence, it is a process of authenticity that involves the whole person or one's whole being in the world and not just relative to our freedom in the world. How we reflect on our thoughts and actions to empathise with others also assists us with our meaning making endeavours. It is interesting to note that each existential theorist has themselves lived through life struggles, which is further suggestive that existential thought is not just an academic consideration but is in fact incumbent with reflections made upon life challenges that have been faced.

Søren Kierkegaard

Søren Kierkegaard is often referred to as the founder of existential philosophy. His writings discuss choice and commitment and individuality, he placed much of his attention on considering how individuals emotionally manage major life events. We can identify with this when we consider the multitude of decisions individuals and families must make about palliative care choices and end of life directives. Individuals and families can feel supported by their faith in these times, whereas others can feel at odds. In response to this differentiation, Kierkgaard suggests that without questioning, we have no faith. We do not require faith to understand issues or items of tangibility. But as humans we can find ourselves in places where we have an inner need for it, especially if we need to have a belief in something that there is little evidence of support for. In other words, our human need for faith is evident when placed in a situation whereby there is a significant level of uncertainty or doubt.

A 'leap of faith' stems from Kierkegaard's writings. For example, it is expected that an individual will fear the uncertainty of death and it is commonplace that the uncertainty experienced will lead to a need to strengthen faith rather than lose it. We cannot know how we will deal with facing our own death until we are facing it, nothing can be alluded to, until we are in that place (Walsh, 2018).

Friedrich Nietzsche

Friedrich Nietzsche is famous for his writing around the concept of nihilism, or existential nihilism – the idea that there are times whereby life can be perceived to have no meaning or purpose. Individuals in palliative or more focused end of life care can experience existential nihilism and think that their life has been meaningless or that there is no longer any reason for them to live. For Nietzsche it is not meaning or happiness that drives us in our lives but 'will to power', achievement and reaching an enviable life positioning. From this position, we can reason that for individuals who have been high achievers in life, once they become seriously ill, they will struggle to see purpose in their lives. We cannot rule out that if this happens it could be because there is a level of depression or some other internalising mental health difficulty. However, many great thinkers have supported the concept of existential nihilism or at least they struggle to rule it out of total consideration. Nietzsche's ideas on individuality, morality and the meaning of existence are also said to have influenced the thinking of philosophers Martin Heidegger, Jacques Derrida, and Michel Foucault.

Unfortunately, Nietzsche spent the last ten years of his life in a mental asylum. The reason for his insanity remains unclear with some arguing syphilis and others a brain disease or the overuse of sedatives. Whatever the reason, it is through his illness struggles that he was driven to engage with existential thought. He died in Weimar, Germany on 25 August 1900 (Stegenga, 2018).

Victor Frankl

In opposition to Nietzsche's 'will to power', Victor Frankl (1947/2021) argues that it is our 'will to meaning' which influences human behaviour. His theory details that if we can find meaning in demanding situations, then we will find the strength and will to live through the most terrible of situations.

Frankl described meaningful living as being present in the moment, being focused on life and not on what may or may not be achieved through living. He suggests however, that we are always death aware, and this awareness also adds meaning to our lives. Frankl's theory stems from his experiences and observations from being in World War II Nazi concentration camps. He lived through the hells of starvation, being overworked, living in poor hygienic conditions, and suffering torture. In this time people died through the physical abuse or emotional suffering, giving in to the immeasurable feelings of powerlessness, hopelessness, and despair.

Frankl puts forward the notion that there were characteristic differences between those who lived and those who did not. Those who managed to get through such shocking times were sometimes emotionally stronger, but in general they had got through it by concentrating on another person or event to live for. This purpose to live, gave them life meaning and helped them to battle the desperation urges and to fight death. He suggests that meaning is the essential motivational force of our lives (Frankl, 1947/2021).

The following comprise the basic principles of Frankl's existential theory:

- We are driven to find meaning in our present, even when facing the most difficult conditions.
- We have the freedom to make personal choices in life. These choices can be actioned or not, we are in control of how we react and experience, even if that experience is one of suffering.
- The freedom of choice allows us to claim control and personal responsibility for our decision making.

Frankl writes that we should 'Live as if you were living already for the second time and as if you had acted the first time as wrongly as you are about to act now!' (Frankl, 1947/2021 pp.131–132). With this thinking we can perceive that our past can be altered in the present.

Jean-Paul Sartre

Although not widely discussed Jean-Paul Sartre used barbiturates and amphetamines in his youth and as a result for many years suffered with visual hallucinations. His writings gained attention from 1938 onwards when his first novel 'The somber and anxiety driven nausea' was published. He became recognised as an existentialist when he wrote 'Being and Nothingness' in 1943 where the crux of his work centred on how 'existence precedes essence' (Satre, 2021) and that it is not until we have experienced life, events, and achievements that we can reflect and visualise our 'essence' which is representative of what we have done. At the end of life, individuals may feel they are just existing. Sartre recognises this and suggests that death itself makes us existent only in the outside world, the lived experience of existence is no longer. This is a move from essence to existence which for many can be emotionally difficult to comprehend. However, Sartre also wrote about how it is useful to experience 'death consciousness' (Satre, 2021) so that we can realise the important aspects of life. Individuals who can reflect and find meaning discuss such as being a 'silver lining' to the fact that their death is soon to be. For others, this happening can make them ruminate on time and opportunities lost.

Rollo May

Rollo May like his peers had several negative earlier life experiences, from his parents divorcing, his sister experiencing mental illness to him as an adult then suffering from tuberculosis for two years. In his own search for meaning, he spent time in Greece teaching English and in the summertime, he studied with Alfred Adler. He also was a student at the Union Theological Seminary in New York and befriended Paul Tillich, a Christian Existentialist and then teacher. Whilst ill, he became very anxious and to help alleviate his anxiety he read many works of philosophy and psychology, including those of Kierkegaard, Nietzsche and Freud, and others. These writings resonated with his experience of living with a life-threatening disease. He believed he would die if he did not master his emotional struggles. May started to explore further the concepts of existential crisis and anxiety, writing his articulation of these and the contrasting concepts of meaningfulness of hope, and joy (Eliason et al., 2010). May is critical of western society in his accounts, suggesting that a wealth of western society is spiritually impotent due to the materialistic patterns of behaviour that exist. He argued that especially western individuals need to reconsider their relationship with the world and to also re-evaluate their concept of love (Kiser, 2007).

Frederick Perls

Frederick Perls did not take a direct path to his philosophical writings. He was raised following the Jewish faith in Germany and yet on a number of occasions as a youth he also found himself in trouble with the law. However, he was a determined thinker, eventually becoming a medical doctor and served in the First World War as a medic. Like Frankl, and May, Perls argued that individuals have agency and control and therefore must be rendered as having responsibility for their actions and have the persuasion to alter their lives at any point through their life course. To do this he argued we must understand our selves and our subjective realities (Perls, 1969; Eliason et al., 2010).

Irvin Yalom

Irvin Yalom was born to Russian immigrant parents in 1931 in the USA. He was raised in a segregated area of Washington, DC. Amongst other families also struggling with a day to day poverty existence. Yalom became a keen reader and chose to become a psychiatrist, impassioned by the uniqueness of individuals lived experiences and their willingness to share them with him. Irvin Yalom is responsible for transferring much existential thought relative to psychotherapy into broader thinking. As a result of observing the behaviour of many individuals, he suggests that expressed conflicts are relatable to four key issues:

1. Death – which manifests as the tension between knowing we all must die to musing over our mortality and our desire to continue living.
2. Freedom – this is alarming for many. If we have no direction, we have total responsibility over our lives lived. Distress can result from facing the groundlessness of being and yearning for structure and guidance.
3. Existential isolation – this is about how we can become disconnected from ourselves. Yalom suggests that intrapersonal conflict can ensue from the tension that exists at times where we feel isolated and have an inner need to be part of the larger whole. Death is something we experience in isolation, alone – just as we experience our birth.
4. Meaninglessness – as humans we are programmed to seek meaningfulness and responsible for attributing some sense of meaning to our existence. Distress ensues when we are in a position where we try to find meaning in what feels to be a meaningless situation (May and Yalom, 1989.

Ernesto Spinelli and Robert Neimeyer

Ernesto Spinelli and Robert Neimeyer are contemporary theorists who have tried to broaden and expand existential theory. Spinelli (2005, pp.148–149) in exploring existential phenomenology identified four inter-relational realms of descriptive inquiry that he suggests are required when investigating individual's worldviews:

1. The *I-focused* realm – explores the individual's experience of self in the world.
2. The *you-focused* realm attempts to identify and describe the individual's experience of other in the current encounter. This would include the individual's experience of you the enquirer.
3. The *we-focused* realm explores emerging facets of the experience between individual and enquirer. At this point the individual is in the present moment and processes the experience and its immediacy.
4. The *they-focused* realm of encounter considers relationships that comprise the individual's wider world of others, beyond the enquirer.

Alternatively, Robert Neimeyer combines existentialism with constructivism with his theory of meaning reconstruction. Meaning reconstruction is effective in helping individuals through periods of grieving, loss, and death anxiety. It is our human nature to assign meaning to our encounters and lived experiences and to develop subjective belief systems that emanate from our connectedness to others and our culture. When we experience loss, our constructed belief systems can be challenged, impacting on how we view ourselves in the world and our personal identities. Neimeyer suggested that at such times of conflict there is an opportunity for meaning reconstruction. The use of narrative therapy is key to meaning reconstruction (Neimeyer, 2000a; 2000b, 2020; Neimeyer et al., 2010).

In drawing on the work of these key thinkers within existentialism, we can move away from a mainstream health psychology perspective and explore phenomena in more depth. Looking at the issues themselves as they occur throughout serious illness for children, young people, families, and professionals and to explore the different contexts that provide meaning to an individual's 'suffering' and related experiences.

Chapter summary

Dame Cicely Saunders was a nurse, social worker, and medical doctor whose desire was to build a new area of healthcare that would be focused on providing a quality of life in dying and would support the holistic needs of individuals and families. Following the opening of St Christopher's hospice in the UK and the work of Kubler-Ross whose ethnographical work also identified the needs of dying people in the hospital setting, moved professionals in the USA to accept the need for changing attitudes towards care and the Hospice philosophy was then embraced. The term palliative care was soon born, coined by the Canadian Medic Balfour Mount. United these key scholars brought the topic of the care of the dying onto medical centre stage. Palliative care has since been embraced world-wide with initiatives promoting its continued development and uptake, even in countries where provision is not yet prevalent. The Modern Hospice remains a key element of hospice care provision. Due to people living longer with complexity hospice care is now a provider of specialist palliative care. Throughout a disease trajectory an individual may receive hospital and hospice based palliative care with much of their support emanating from community provisions.

Essential to the care of the dying and intrinsic to the palliative care philosophy regardless of location, is the concept of spirituality. The ultimate question of 'who am I?' is essential to our being regardless of our health status. For many, the drive to make meaning in life is that which defines our contentment and serenity. For others, regrets from the past, exacerbate feelings of hopelessness, emptiness, and dread. With good palliative care, professionals can bear witness to and support suffering, provide compassion and empathy and engage individuals in meaning making interventions. Spirituality is the 'thing' we cannot quite fit into a neat tidy box or definition for all but is that 'thing' which enables us to have an engagement with the meaningfulness of our lives.

For Kirkegaard it is through facing the end of our lives that we reach the place within ourselves whereby we can sit alone in contemplation of our suffering. Frankl (1947/2021) states that 'meaning can be found in life literally up to the last moment, up to the last breath, in the face of death' (p.76). For Yalom it is our personal struggle with death and dying that creates anxiety and the need for support. Our freedom creates choice, responsibility, and guilt. For Heidegger (1996), human existence is never static, death and death anxiety are unique and personally experienced: 'The existential meaning of our ending is utterly personal and must be seized as a grieving, which can constitute our wholeness or potency' (p286).

The isolation of our predicaments can also feel like an ocean that cannot be crossed easily between ourselves and those who matter to us, it can feel meaningless, and it is this meaninglessness that creates our desire as human beings to search for and create personal meaning. Our being towards death thus exposes our ultimate aloneness in the world. For Satre there is no fixed way to be, meaning is created instead through being and existing. In this understanding, a person is defined by what he or she becomes. As Ellin (1995, p. 325) argues, 'giving meaning to your life is something you must do for yourself. And you must do it, as the existentialists quite correctly point out, without any sure proof that what you are doing is correct'.

It is with this philosophical appreciation that we can begin to understand how individuals with palliative care needs and their families continue living with a strength of will and character in the face of adversity, conflict, fear and dying.

Key issues

1. The hospice movement initiated by the work of Saunders stemmed from her interest in the holistic care of individuals facing shortened lives and how pain was not just physical it was existential.
2. By providing holistic care to the dying, we encounter their physical, psychological, social and spiritual needs.
3. Delivered by generalist and specialist teams, palliative care provision for children and young people can now be found in community and inpatient settings, continually evolving to meet the needs of the growing populations of individuals with life limiting/threatening conditions and their families. This is evident in how hospice provision now is considered as specialist provision supporting those who require specialist palliative care due to the complexity of their conditions. There can be debate however, as to what conditions and stages of disease trajectories and indeed what symptoms, may constitute complexity.
4. Regardless of where and how palliative care is provided, holistic care and support is offered and often spiritual needs and a supportive stance towards an individual and families spirituality is required by providers/health and social care professionals. Existentialist philosophy identifies that we as human beings are universally characterised by our concern for meaning and purpose and this is heightened when we are faced with a serious illness and shortened life prognosis.

Box 1.1 Reflective Questions

1. If palliative care is a philosophy of care, do we need a designated palliative care sector of healthcare for children and young people?
2. Is your interest in palliative care influenced by your own witnessing of suffering?

References

Bultz, B. and Butow, P., 2011. *Handbook of communication in oncology and palliative care.* Oxford University Press.

Breitbart, W, Poppito S, Rosenfeld B, et al., 2012. Pilot randomized controlled trial of individual meaning-centered psychotherapy for patients with advanced cancer. *Journal of Clinical Oncology*, *30*(12), pp.1304–1309.

Calanzani, N., Higginson, I.J., and Gomes, B., 2013. *Current and future needs for hospice care: an evidence-based report.* Help The Hospices Commission into the future of hospice care.

Chater, M., 2020. *Reforming Religious Education: Power and Knowledge in a Worldviews Curriculum.* John Catt Educational.

Chater, M.F., 2000. Spirituality as struggle: poetics, experience, and the place of the spiritual in educational encounter. *International Journal of Children's Spirituality*, *5*(2), pp.193–201.

Chochinov, H.M., 2012. *Dignity therapy: Final words for final days*. OUP USA.

Clark, D. and Seymour, J., 1999. *Reflections on palliative care*. The Open University Press.

Clark, D., Stillion, J.M. and Attig, T., 2015. Hospice care of the dying. *Death, dying, and bereavement: Contemporary perspectives, institutions, and practices*, 96–148. Springer.

Craven, J. and Wald, F.S., 1975. Hospice care for dying patients. *The American Journal of Nursing*, *75*(1), pp.1816–1822.

Dictionary, O.E., 2018. Hospice.

Dossey, L., 2014. Spirituality and nonlocal mind: A necessary dyad. *Spirituality in Clinical Practice*, *1*(1), p.29.

Dos Santos, F.C., Macieira, T.G., Yao, Y., Hunter, S., Madandola, O.O., Cho, H., Bjarnadottir, R.I., Dunn Lopez, K., Wilkie, D.J. and Keenan, G.M., 2022. Spiritual Interventions Delivered by Nurses to Address Patients' Needs in Hospitals or Long-Term Care Facilities: A Systematic Review. *Journal of Palliative Medicine*, *25*(4), pp.662–677.

Eliason, G.T., Samide, J.L., Williams, G. and Lepore, M.F., 2010. Existential theory and our search for spirituality. *Journal of Spirituality in Mental Health*, *12*(2), pp. 86–111.

Ellin J (1995) *Morality and the meaning of life: an introduction to ethical theory*. Harcourt Brace.

EPICC Network: Enhancing nurses and midwives' competence in providing spiritual care through innovative education and compassionate care. https://blogs.staffs.ac.uk/epicc/ (accessed 22 May 2022).

Frankl, V.E., 1947/2021. *Man's search for meaning*. Simon and Schuster.

Henderson, J., Horden, P. and Pastore, A. eds., 2007. *The impact of Hospitals, 300–2000*. Peter Lang.

Hospice UK (2022) www.hospiceuk.org/latest-from-hospice-uk/hospice-uk-responds-funding-hospice-sector (accessed 25 May 2022).

Heidegger, M. (1996) *Being and time* (J. Stambaugh, Trans.). State University of New York Press.

Hindmarch, T., Dalrymple, J., Smith, M. and Barclay, S., 2022. Spiritual interventions for cancer pain: a systematic review and narrative synthesis. *BMJ Supportive & Palliative Care*, *12*(1), pp.1–9.

Kiser, S., 2007. Sacred dialectic: The centrality of paradox in the worldview of Rollo May. *The Humanistic Psychologist*, *35*(2), p.191.

Kübler-Ross, E., 2009. *Death: The final stage*. Simon and Schuster.

May, R. and Yalom, I., 1989. Existential psychotherapy. *Current Psychotherapies* (10th Edition), Edited by: Wedding, D. and Corsini, R.J. (2014) pp.363–402. Brooks/Cole.

Montross-Thomas, L.P., Joseph, J., Edmonds, E.C., Palinkas, L.A. and Jeste, D.V., 2018. Reflections on wisdom at the end of life: qualitative study of hospice patients aged 58–97 years. *International Psychogeriatrics*, *30*(12), pp.1759–1766.

Neimeyer, R.A. 2000a. 'The language of loss: Grief therapy as a process of meaning reconstruction'. In *Meaning reconstruction and the experience of loss*, Edited by: Neimeyer, R.A. 261–292. American Psychological Association.

Neimeyer, R.A. 2000b. Searching for the meaning of meaning: Grief therapy and the process of reconstruction *Death Studies*, *24*, pp. 541–558.

Neimeyer, R.A., 2020. What's new in meaning reconstruction?: Advancing grief theory and practice. *Grief Matters: The Australian Journal of Grief and Bereavement*, *23*(1), pp.4–9.

Neimeyer, R.A., Burke, L.A., Mackay, M.M., and van Dyke Stringer, J.G., 2010. Grief therapy and the reconstruction of meaning: From principles to practice. *Journal of Contemporary Psychotherapy*, *40*(2), pp.73–83.

Park, C.L., Sherman, A.C., Jim, H.S. and Salsman, J.M., 2015. Religion/spirituality and health in the context of cancer: Cross-domain integration, unresolved issues, and future directions. *Cancer*, *121*(21), pp.3789–3794.

Parkinson, J. (2015) How hospices care for the dying. www.bbc.co.uk/news/magazine-34452836 (accessed 25 May 2022).

Perls, F.S., 1969. Gestalt therapy verbatim

Puchalski, C., Jafari, N., Buller, H., Haythorn, T., Jacobs, C. and Ferrell, B. (2020). Interprofessional spiritual care education curriculum: A milestone toward the provision of spiritual care. *Journal of Palliative Medicine*, *23*(6), pp.777–784.

Rego, F. and Nunes, R. (2019). The interface between psychology and spirituality in palliative care. *Journal of Health Psychology*, *24*(3), pp.279–287.

Rosa, W.E., Chochinov, H.M., Coyle, N., Hadler, R.A. and Breitbart, W.S., 2022. Attending to the existential experience in oncology: dignity and meaning amid awareness of death. *JCO Global Oncology*, *8*, pp.e2200038.

Salsman, J.M., Pustejovsky, J.E., Jim, H.S., Munoz, A.R., Merluzzi, T.V., George, L., Park, C.L., Danhauer, S.C., Sherman, A.C., Snyder, M.A. and Fitchett, G., 2015. A meta-analytic approach to examining the correlation between religion/spirituality and mental health in cancer. *Cancer*, *121*(21), pp.3769–3778.

Sartre, J.P., 2021. Existentialism is a Humanism. In *Existentialism is a Humanism*, 17–72. Yale University Press.

Saunders, C., 1965. The last stages of life. *The American Journal of Nursing*, *65*(3), pp.70–75.

Sherman, A.C., Merluzzi, T.V., Pustejovsky, J.E., Park, C.L., George, L., Fitchett, G., Jim, H.S., Munoz, A.R., Danhauer, S.C., Snyder, M.A. and Salsman, J.M., 2015. A meta-analytic review of religious or spiritual involvement and social health among cancer patients. *Cancer*, *121*(21), pp.3779–3788.

Sister Frances BBC media article, November (2009): www.bbc.co.uk/berkshire/content/articles/2009/01/09/helen_house_feature.shtml

Spinelli, E. 2005. *The interpreted world: An introduction to phenomenological psychology*, Sage Publications.

Stegenga, J., 2018. *Medical nihilism*. Oxford University Press.

Syme, A. and Bruce, A., 2009. Hospice and palliative care: What unites us, what divides us? *Journal of Hospice & Palliative Nursing*, *11*(1), pp.19–24.

Tobin, R.S., Cosiano, M.F., O'Connor, C.M., Fiuzat, M., Granger, B.B., Rogers, J.G., Tulsky, J.A., Steinhauser, K.E. and Mentz, R.J., 2022. *Spirituality in Patients with Heart Failure*. JACC: Heart Failure.

TfSL (2012) 'guidance for children's end of life care' TfSL (accessed 20 May, 2022)

Walsh, S., 2018. *Kierkegaard and religion: Personality, character, and virtue*. Cambridge University Press.

2 Children and young people's palliative care needs

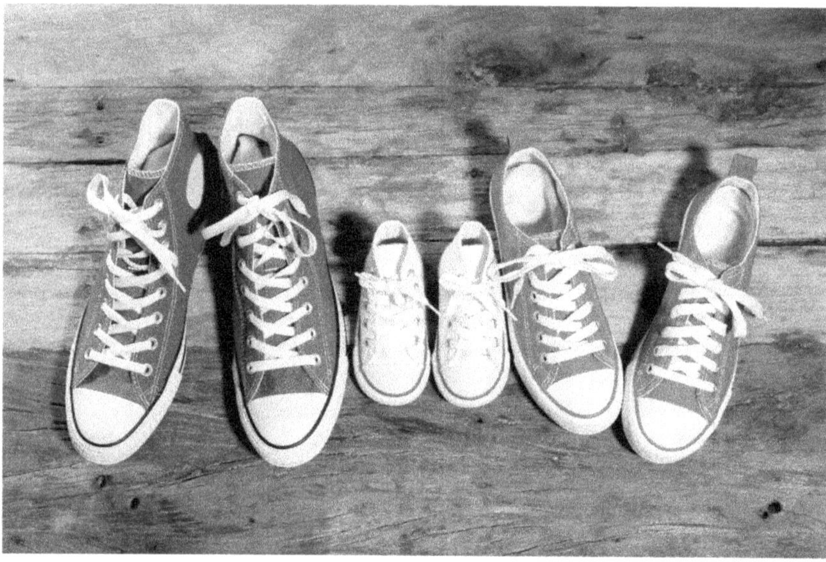

Figure 2.1 A photograph of three different sized shoes.
Sourced from Shutterstock images.

Introduction

Palliative care addresses the holistic needs of individuals across the lifespan. In taking a lifespan approach to understanding palliative care needs, we also acknowledge that individual and developmental needs are entwined and embedded within socio-ecological contexts. The experience of palliative care is lived in response to the integration of developmental needs and the developmental tasks that occur for individuals amidst social, institutional, and cultural factors. This chapter highlights what we know about age and developmental related differences in terms of illness and death understanding and palliative

DOI: 10.4324/9781003340287-3

care support needs – at person and family centred levels where needed. The chapter starts with a consideration of neonatal palliative care and the types of conditions that meet the criteria for palliative support pre and post birth. Then continues with the palliative care considerations and challenges for children and adolescents, emerging and young adults.

Neonatal palliative care

In 2020, 2,226 infant deaths were recorded (ONS, 2022). Each year there are infant deaths where families would benefit from the support of a palliative care team prior to birth. There are also dedicated perinatal palliative care teams within neonatal medicine who support families where infants are diagnosed with serious illness antenatally.

Palliative care provision for infants is family centred, meaning support is also extended to key family members. Each family has different dynamics, some will include support from grandparents for example, where others might include support from significant others without kinship. When there are many uncertainties with an infant's diagnosis and prognosis the palliative care team will aim to achieve quality contact time between the infant and their family immediately following birth, leading up to and following the death of the infant. Spending time with families also helps professionals to negotiate who should be included in the discussions about care options and support. This support can be emotionally intensive for both families and professionals. However, it is important that the multidisciplinary team can understand and accommodate the cultural and spiritual needs of each family, which again can be diverse. Families in these situations receive dedicated support in the neonatal intensive care unit (NICU). Providing palliative care within the confined space of the NICU is also challenging as space and privacy is limited. The conceptual framework underpinning neonatal palliative care is summarised in Figure 2.2.

The perinatal palliative care pathway (Together for Short Lives, 2017) details four condition categories that meet palliative care access requirements for infants:

Box 2.1 Condition categories that meet palliative care access requirements for infants (TfSL, 2017):

1 **Life-threatening conditions where curative treatment may be feasible but can fail**

Involving palliative care is supportive for infants where treatment has failed or may fail. It may be the case that the child later responds well to treatment and becomes stable with the potential to thrive. In which case palliative care services would then no longer be needed.

Examples of conditions: extreme prematurity, congenital heart disease, severe PPHN

2 **Conditions where premature death is inevitable**

Intensive treatment and care delivered to prolong life and allow participation activities.

Examples of conditions: chromosomal abnormalities, bilateral renal agenesis

3 **Progressive conditions without curative treatment options**

Treatment is exclusively palliative, there is no hope for a cure but the treatment may span months or years.

Examples of conditions: spinal muscular atrophy, mitochondrial disorders

4 **Irreversible but non-progressive conditions causing severe disability, leading to susceptibility to health complications and likelihood of premature death**

Examples of conditions: severe hypoxic ischaemic encephalopathy

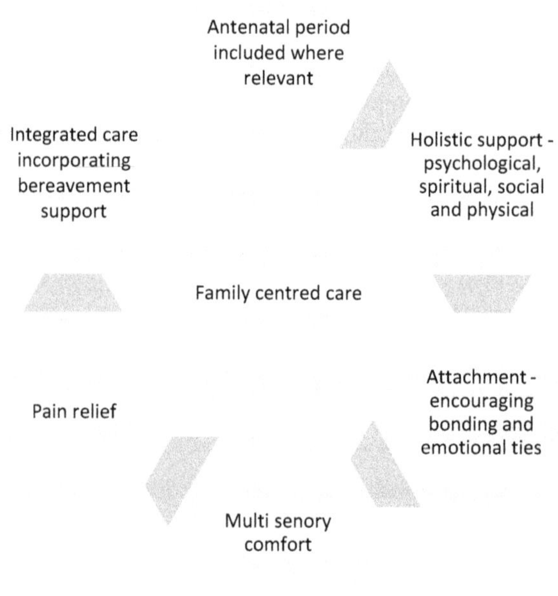

Figure 2.2 The conceptual framework underpinning neonatal palliative care. Adapted from Balaguer et al., 2012.

There are infants who will require most of their support in intensive care but there are also infants, as we can see from the categories above, that will live beyond their time needed in the NICU. Decisions will then be made relating to prognosis as to what further cares may be provided within the hospital setting, hospice or at home.

Comfort care

As noted, where possible palliative care is offered to families before birth. However, the reality is that for most infants receiving palliative care (at least in the UK), palliative care and support will have commenced following birth and often after intensive care support has been withdrawn. This means that the infant is likely to be sedated and receiving pain relief intravenously. These medical actions are taken to try to ensure that the infant is comfortable. It is difficult to ascertain an infant's experiences of pain especially when they are born extremely prematurely. There are scales that can be used to assess pain responses and evidence shows that pain medication does decrease these visible pain signs in infants. In times of uncertainty, however, it is still usually advised that the infant does receive sedation and pain relief. This care runs alongside nonmedical orientated comfort interventions including skin to skin and kangaroo care, using techniques that provide infants with positive touch and positioning with family care givers.

Other simple interventions are also helpful, including administering sucrose and comfort holding. Feeding is also important and can provide comfort. Just giving tiny amounts of feed is part of comfort care. Of course, if the infant is expected to live beyond time in the NICU then scheduled feeding plans would need to be orchestrated and be relevant to the infant's condition needs (Bidegain and Younge, 2015).

End of life care

Reorienting care and explaining to families that care is now palliative is difficult. Clear communication about the situation needs to be conveyed to families and explanations provided as to why ventilator or other supports will be removed. The end-of-life process in NICU also involves the removal of the endotracheal tube. This is otherwise referred to as compassionate extubation (Donoho et al., 2021). Families need to know why it is kind to the infant to take these actions and be offered information so that they are prepared for how the infant will respond. Parents especially will be engulfed in sadness and fear about the proximity of their child's death. If this is a certain outcome, they may need further explanation as to why there is no longer hope for cure or for extending life without suffering. Not all infants respond in the same way, so it is important to explain there is uncertainty. Sometimes infants will gasp or breathe without support, they may indeed continue to live for hours and sometimes days after extubation. Professionals will need to talk through the array of changes including colour change so that parents can feel less frightened when it happens (Needle, 2010).

An infant death in the neonatal period is difficult for families to accept. Often families are already grieving for a loss of a 'normal' pregnancy if their child has arrived very early. The medical and life sustaining interventions the infant receives can also make the bonding process more difficult for parents. As much time as possible needs to be afforded for families to be with their babies and support provided for them to engage in memory making activities. The memory making can support them through the grieving process. Although the infant's life has been short there are still memories of joy that can be reflected upon. Engagement in these activities with families can also strengthen relationships between professionals and families, which benefits openness and trust if tough decisions later need to be made. Photographs and videos, clothes and other materials used throughout NICU can complement the reflecting and storying that families might want to engage with.

Culturally appropriate care is always needed and a key focus of family centred care. Staff on NICU are provided with training around diverse cultural practices around death and bereavement. Cultural awareness in this context can also help health care professionals to appreciate family norms with respect to care of the infant's body following death. Some level of awareness is important, but this does not remove the need to also speak with families about their wishes.

Palliative care for children and adolescents

Children and adolescents can require palliative care that is much more varied than that for infants and adults, not least due to the nuances of the many different conditions they can be experiencing. Hain et al. (2013) did an analysis of death certificates and determined that in the UK alone there had been 376 conditions requiring children's palliative care. Some of these conditions are limited to childhood, and may be rare, complex to understand and manage due to unknown disease trajectories.

The population of children, adolescents, and young adults with serious illness is growing not least due to medical and technological advances, which means that it is now possible to live longer with life-limiting conditions. UK data has determined that 66.4 per 10,000 individuals from 0 to 19 years were living with life-limiting conditions in 2017, with prevalence forecasted to increase to 84.2 per 10,000 by 2030 (Fraser et al., 2021). However, even in the UK where palliative care is more developed than in many other countries for children and young people, it is estimated that only 18.6% of these young people in 2016 with serious illness were in receipt of palliative care before their death (Widger et al., 2016). A further study identified that where palliative care was received, those who chose to die in a hospital or hospice setting were supported to do so. However, just 58% of young people with cancer conditions died at home after they had stated it was their place of preference for their death (Stillwell et al., 2020). Increasingly we are aware that providing palliative care early in a disease trajectory can improve quality of life and symptom control outcomes. This thinking also encourages supported advanced care planning and promotes a choice in the place of death (PoD) outside of hospital; if discussions are had in advance of the individual's close proximity to death, then it is easier to action individuals' wishes and for health and social care professionals to put support in place for families (Mitchell et al., 2017).

In resource rich countries we benefit from advances in modern day medicine to sustain and extend life. As such, accepting a no treatment option is difficult for health care professionals to contend and is increasingly at odds with western thinking synonymous with preserving life and increasing longevity. The psychological processes and related emotional turmoil that individuals and families go through when there is a transition from curative to solely palliative care is hard to envisage and perhaps more so when the individual is a child. Families can struggle with communicating with their children about the serious illness and its ultimate trajectory. The isolation of no communication about prognosis and end of life is discussed by Bluebond-Langner (1978/2020) in her seminal work with seriously ill children. Children may vicariously learn about their eventuality from listening to conversations or experiencing the loss of their peers. Dependent on the age of the child and their mental/cognitive capacity, they can have a great fear of death, and more so they can have major concerns around the separation from their parents or peers. Separation is emotionally difficult and impactful on normative developmental tasks for children and young people.

Living with a life limiting/threatening condition can be particularly challenging for adolescents. At a time where adolescents hold much attention on their external image, they are confronted with changes in body image or the increasing realisation that they are different to their peers. Their privacy needs cannot always be achieved and although we appreciate that adolescents can be easily embarrassed at showing their bodies, they are confronted with needing to be reliant on others for intimate cares. Through this phase of development adolescents are also dealing with changing relationships with their parents and siblings, striving for a little more distance and independence, less familial intimacy, but with a desire now for romantic relationships. These needs can be more difficult to satisfy when the young person is limited in their movement and communication or is unable to be autonomous and live day to day without supervision. Where adolescents can understand their situation, it is advocated that to limit trauma they need to be involved in decision making about their current and future needs (DeCourcey et al., 2019).

As suggested by Julie Stokes, founder of Winston's Wish (a leading charity that offers support to children facing anticipatory grief and bereavement), in resource rich countries we are not comfortable with children being sad. We also know that children become aware of situations and without any adult support they can get things wrong, get sadder and feel more alone. Therefore, where possible and not withstanding family preferences, information should be provided to children that is truthful but provided in a format they can understand and is delivered at their pace. Children facing a shortened life prognosis need to know that they will always be in receipt of care and that they can also be involved in their care choices. Although they will be sad once the truth is told or reinforced by the telling, as compared to adults we see that children can have the capacity to cope well. Older children and adolescents also welcome time alone with health and social care professionals. In these times and away from families they may find they can better find their voice and share their thoughts and wishes (Mallon, 2018).

Family centred care

Involving families in supporting and caring for their children with palliative care needs is a necessity of good practice. Although serious illness can impact autonomy, some life limiting, and life-threatening conditions do not impact cognition and related capacity until the end of life. Therefore, as young people grow and become more autonomous, their decision-making capacity also changes. While children and younger adolescents need the involvement of parents and siblings, older adolescents may prioritise significant others, and friends in assisting with decision making. It can often be difficult to balance the needs and desires of all members of a family but treating the young person as an equal and providing advice or assistance for them to make their own decisions enables independence, self-confidence, and a sense of self. To the best of an individual's ability, children and adolescents should be encouraged to share in decision making with caregivers to consider the wishes of the individual as best as possible (DeCourcey et al., 2019; Jacobs et al., 2014).

Cultural and spiritual needs

The experience of palliative care for children and adolescents can be influenced by their cultural heritage including their religion, ethnicity, socio economic status, education level, gender, and sexuality. These issues can also impact on their decision making and their families decision making around their serious illness and treatment and care options, especially when it comes to advanced care planning and end of life care. It is normative, for young people to begin reflecting on and developing their belief and value systems and it is possible that their views and perceptions will hold some difference to those of their family. This is where health and social care professionals can act to engage young people in discussions and activities to expose their wishes and for them then to mediate with families to ensure the young person's wishes are met (Alvarez et al., 2017; Roeland et al., 2019).

Most serious illnesses bring with them psychological impacts for young people, to be dealt with alongside the physical challenges. As a result, communication between health and social care professionals and young people is paramount, not least to be able to assess the young person's needs and provide supportive intervention where necessary. A substantial proportion of young people with life shortening prognoses want to know how much time they may have left and to be involved in related care discussions. These conversations can impact on their quality of life and end of life care choices. In making these decisions young people will frequently consider their family's needs too. In situations where families are unaware of their needs, the young person can suffer heightened levels of anxiety and poor psychosocial adjustment. There can also be more difficulties in regulating pain management and reports of feeling isolated. If there is a discord of communication, families will also experience more distress (Sansom-Daly et al., 2020).

Psychological needs at the end of life

The psychological needs of children and young people as they live toward the end of their lives are wide ranging. They can be prevented from undertaking normative developmental tasks, for example, attending school and forming meaningful friendships. Feeling behaviourally restricted can impact both their behavioural and emotional functioning. Fears can be crippling as children and young people approach the very end of life, including the fear of death and the fear of pain. A deep sadness, anxiety and loneliness can be prevalent in the final weeks of life. Where possible, an interdisciplinary team can work together to alleviate these symptoms, adopting interventions to support the individual and family. In addition, it has been realised that where children and young people are struggling to connect face to face with peers, that social media is an excellent tool of communication for them. They can connect via blogs, Instagram and facebook pages, twitter feeds and chat rooms with peers experiencing the same symptoms or living with the same or other life hindering serious illnesses. Being able to make connections with peers on similar journeys can enhance self-efficacy, feelings of being in control, and coping (Graetz et al., 2019; Perales et al., 2016).

Any negative psychological symptoms can also be explained by the anticipatory grief process they are going through. This grief experience can influence concerns for mental health but can also lead to a point of acceptance.

Transition

Children and young people have started living longer with their serious illnesses, and as a result we are now seeing greater numbers of young people being transferred to adult services. There are still some young adults who will be supported by children and young people's hospice care into their mid or late twenties, sometimes beyond, but because of the total population of young people with palliative care needs increasing, there is a push to transfer young people to adult services once they reach adulthood.

However, it was realised in the mid-1990s that it was too great a leap for young people to move directly to adult care services on reaching adulthood. Having been supported by children's services to then be moved directly to adult care services with vastly different models of care, and with different teams of health and social care professionals was felt to be a further burden on wellbeing for individuals and families. With more responsibility on the young adult and their family to negotiate all their cares in a less supported fashion, there is a risk of poorer outcomes. Such moves can also be affected by deteriorating physical health and/or capacity. Instead, and where possible, it is realised that there needs to be a supported move and dedicated young adult services that can lay as a middle ground or transition period between child and adult care services (Knighting, et al. 2018; Mennito and Clark, 2010).

Transition has been defined as 'The purposeful, planned process that addresses the medical, psychosocial and educational/vocational needs of young people and young adults with chronic physical and medical conditions as they move from child-centred to adult-oriented healthcare systems' (Rosen, 2003). Kirk and Fraser (2014) however, highlighted the following difficulties in transition for young people with palliative care needs:

- There is a lack of multi-agency arrangements and co-ordination between services
- A dearth of key workers for individuals and families
- Different services have different adult criteria for support
- Adult services do not provide the level of contact or support that children's services do
- There are fewer disease specialists in adult services
- Schools are no longer involved in service provision
- There is a vastly different culture of care
- There is less tailored support for holistic issues
- Relationships with children's service providers break down.

In recognition of these difficulties young adult focused care models and facilities have been developed. Most notably, young adults are now recognised as a distinct group and vulnerable. In some areas, there are now systems in place for better child and adult service collaboration and supportive interventions in place to help young adults build their own care teams to suit their palliative care and developmental needs (Clark and Fasciano, 2015). There remains however work to be done to provide the continuity of care and specialist respite care for young adults that is afforded by children's services.

Continued developmental needs through adulthood

The developmental stages of young adulthood through to middle age are times of intimacy resulting in the emotional and physical commitment to social, educational, career, partner, and dependent affiliations (Erikson, 1968). Those living with serious illness have many complexities to navigate alongside their 'patient' identity. Relationships are evolving but independence can be skewed by their needed dependence on others.

Physical needs

These are the years of peak sexual development; however, disease and treatment impacts can mean that there are continued influences of physiology including influences on hormone regulation that can also affect growth. Any anticipated difficulties or changes should be points of discussion and supported by ongoing informational support. Adults can also experience greater symptom burden, due to the nature of the disease and the longer end stage periods now seen in some life limiting and life-threatening conditions. This can mean more treatment therapies and higher pharmacological doses (Levine et al., 2017).

Cognitive needs

Brain development has been demonstrated to continue through to the late twenties (Blakemore and Choudhury, 2006; Foulkes, and Blakemore, 2018). Increased connections between regions of the brain, myelination, and synaptic pruning especially in the prefrontal cortex have been seen on imaging of the young adult brain. These changes result in increased executive functioning and abstract thinking including greater skills in calibration of risk and reward, problem solving, prioritising, planning, self-evaluation, and regulation of emotions. Young adults living with serious illness often struggle with the complexities and nuances of medical decision making, however adults with serious illnesses moving into their middle age can struggle with the same complexities, as the presences of illness and the effects of treatment may inhibit brain function and can also regress the individual to have more childlike or inflexible styles of thinking. This can induce greater difficulties in coping with uncertainty and deciding upon care and treatment options. However, the use of a young adult-directed end-of-life care discussion readiness tool followed by the completion of the young adult version of The Five Wishes, Voicing My Choices, has been documented to be effective in the early young adult population (Weiner et al., 2015). Using a readiness tool, to help with the challenging conversations to be had with adults can also help health and social care professionals to appreciate the adults' unique difficulties and lived experiences and work together with the individual to address their goals of care and provide them with reassurance that they are remaining in control of their situation. For those who are too cognitively compromised to continue making decisions then support is given to key family members who are relied upon to maintain the best interests of the adult with serious illness (Sue, et al., 2019).

Psychological needs

As adults refine their self-identity, they also perfect their abilities to understand their own emotions and how they can best relate to others. There can be some emotional instability in young adult years whilst these refinement processes are worked out. As a result, there is a high prevalence of mental health disorders in young adults as compared to other age groups. These include control disorders, eating disorders and substance abuse. Unfortunately, these issues can pervade adult years with then also the added risk of more severe and enduring conditions such as depression and schizophrenia. Not surprisingly, death hastening measures are prevalent amongst the adult population with serious illness. As such it is imperative that specialist mental health support is available via the interdisciplinary team for adults in receipt of palliative care (Hinrichs, et al., 2022; Zebrack et al., 2013).

Social needs

Through adulthood we aim to achieve our life goals, these are often relevant to education and career and relationships. Redefining relationships within our birth families and planning to grow our own families are also normative social developmental tasks. Through adulthood we have economic responsibility and involvement in various communities, at individual and family levels and responsibility for the planning of others, for example our children or partners. However, as serious illness advances, our independence can become strained, and our goals may become harder to achieve. Palliative care teams then need to step in to help individuals modify their goals and help the family find ways to support the individual to still be involved in adult social tasks. Where adults are struggling with issues of identity and feeling a sense of a loss, they should be encouraged to connect with others to help them to relate to others and empathise with others, to engage them in a different type of purpose and by doing so feel supported in their own journey (Bandeali et al., 2020; Reith and Payne, 2009).

Spiritual needs

A serious illness may lead to adults and their families experiencing existential and spiritual concerns. These can relate to perceptions around loss of meaning or purpose in life, a sense of hopelessness, isolation, and fear of dying. Experiences of existential and spiritual suffering can influence the adult to re-evaluate their lives. This can mean a rewriting of the life story in a search for meaning and connectedness because of the disruptive experience of vulnerability. Story telling can lead to change, to self-discovery and meaning making (Anbeek, 2017).

Despite growing recognition of the importance of spiritual care and support in palliative care, this area of care is still the least developed in terms of any formal provision. This can mean that adults with serious illness can live with unmet spiritual needs. Although adults may tell the health and social care professionals involved in their care that they want to talk about these issues, there may be little response to support or refer because of a lack of training and confidence with supporting these types of issues. However, when spiritual needs are not supported this gives rise to spiritual distress and other impacts on more global measures of wellbeing (Damen, et al., 2021; Sinclair and Chochinov, 2012).

The following tables (2.1–2.5) highlight some of the more general palliative care considerations for people at different ages/stages of development. It is recognised that different serious illnesses can render individuals to have different developmental/cognitive abilities than may be expected normatively of their chronological age.

The needs of those receiving palliative care at any life stage are met by expanding expertise and a broadening understanding of individual and family needs. Palliative care is a team effort and requires a combination of skills to facilitate voices, independence, physical comfort and tailored interdisciplinary support for psycho-social and spiritual needs.

Table 2.1 Developmental and palliative care considerations for infants

Developmental phase	*Normative tasks*	*Challenges of palliative care*	*Supportive strategies/ techniques/ considerations*
Infancy	Attachment, language development, achieve fine motor skills, development of sense of self, emotional and body regulation.	Fear of separation from loved ones, becoming avoidant of touch because of painful procedures, disruption of routines, coping with unfamiliar environments, loss of developmental milestones.	Focus is on the needs of parents and the individual's attachment needs. Comfort care. Finding resources for respite care for caregivers. Encourage the family to pre plan for funeral and other end of life decisions if death is expected in infancy. - Encourage creation of memorial items, footprint, lock of hair etc. - Provide education on dying process, in accordance with client's level of readiness. Assess and explore spiritual and cultural beliefs and needs.

Table 2.2 Developmental and palliative care considerations for children

Developmental phase	*Normative tasks*	*Challenges of palliative care*	*Supportive strategies/ techniques/ considerations*
Childhood	Peer development; increasing independence from family; language, concept, and motor development; self-esteem development; creation of positive body image, learning how to act in groups and educational environments.	Conceptual understanding of palliative care and of dying/ shortened life. Fear of separation, isolation from peers, coping with medical treatments, being treated as a 'normal' child at home and school, maintaining a sense of independence.	Involve in treatment decisions appropriate to individual's level of understanding and in accordance with their level of readiness. If given permission, educate school personnel/other social supports. Encourage expression of feelings through creative means, play, art etc. Establish safe places where the individual does not have to receive invasive procedures, be 'different', etc. Provide education on dying process to the individuals level of understanding and readiness. Assess and explore spiritual and cultural beliefs and needs.

Chapter summary

The need for palliative care may be realised antenatally, at the 20-week anomaly scan or may not be apparent until after the baby is born. The role of the NICU is both to care for the infant, providing comfort, minimising distress and managing symptoms and to support the parents and wider family in the tough decisions which may need to be made and the distressing times which may arise. At each chronological stage of life there is a developmental stage with psychosocial and spiritual dimensions for health and social care professionals to work with. All individuals with serious illness experience a series of losses as their illness advances. These losses are felt differently at each developmental stage. Where there is much neurological degeneration through the course of an illness and indeed where the serious illness prevents normative cognitive

Table 2.3 Developmental and palliative care considerations for adolescents

Developmental phase	*Normative tasks*	*Challenges of palliative care*	*Supportive strategies/ techniques/ considerations*
Adolescence	Independence from family, developing a sense of identity, learning how to interact with the other/ preferred sex, developing a positive sense of self and body, coping with the changes associated with puberty, exploring sexuality, developing future plans and goals.	Understanding the disease and treatments, loss of peers, coping with disruptions in physical development, dealing with absences and re -entries into school, feeling physically unattractive (e.g., hair loss), planning for a curtailed future, loss of functions.	Encourage continued involvement in adolescent activities, as tolerated. With permission, offer education to peers, school personnel and other social supports to minimise withdrawal based on fears. Involve adolescent in treatment and care decisions. Encourage expression of feelings through creative means, art, prose, music, etc. Provide education on dying process. Assess and explore spiritual and cultural beliefs and needs.

development, expertise is needed to understand the developmental needs of the individual and family and to consider their related psycho-social and spiritual needs to enable all to live their lives to their fullest. Individuals' needs and families' reactions are entwined and therefore a person and family focus to care is required. The therapeutic value of listening empathetically to 'the story' of children or young people and families is never underestimated by health and social care professionals who need to gain insight into issues of coping, cultural, and spiritual needs, to be able to then fathom what better avenues of supportive care should be offered to individuals and families. Good palliative care is developmentally aware, able to support varied cognitive abilities, can acknowledge and treat symptom burden relative to illness and developmental needs, and promotes times of psychological and spiritual growth, empowering, and honouring individuals with serious illness. This is achieved in drawing on the expertise and skills of professionals with different disciplinary backgrounds, and specialist training in the palliative care team.

Table 2.4 Developmental and palliative care considerations for young adults

Developmental phase	*Normative tasks*	*Challenges of palliative care*	*Supportive strategies/ techniques/ considerations*
Young adulthood	Crystallisation of an identity, developing intimate relationships, setting up own household, educational pursuits leading to career development, contending with transitions in personal, educational, and occupational pursuits, starting a family.	Maintaining intimacy and sexuality, finding one's place in the adult world with a threatened future, continuing in career development, coping with educational and job disruption, contending with increased dependency, coping with urging 'not to give up', concerns with family planning. Loss of functions.	Encourage conversations regarding advance directives. Facilitate group meetings for family and other social supports to minimise potential conflicts and maximise understanding. Provide education on dying process. Provide support and education for sexual intimacy, if faced with physical limitations. Assess and explore spiritual and cultural beliefs and needs.

Key issues

1. Palliative care is offered to individuals across the life span with serious illness and advancing disease.
2. Palliative care for different age groups recognises developmentally appropriate care is required to meet the general care needs of both individual and family.
3. Person and family centred care are approaches to palliative care across the lifespan.
4. Palliative care may begin for infants prior to birth. Palliative care teams support infants and families in the neonatal setting, promoting attachment, memory making and comfort cares.
5. Children and young people prioritise peer support and interaction but still want to be able to have openness with their families for their treatment goals and care needs to be met. This can be a challenge for individuals, families, and health care professionals.

Table 2.5 Developmental and palliative care considerations for adults

Developmental phase	*Normative tasks*	*Challenges of palliative care*	*Supportive strategies/ techniques/ considerations*
Middle age	Developing a sense of generativity in work and personal relationships, potentially taking care of young/ adolescent children and elderly parents, integrating a shifting perspective on the developmental timeline and associated re-evaluation of the self, planning for retirement.	Coping with the dying of peers and parents, developing legacies or aspects of the self of lasting value, making treatment decisions for self or others, concerns with financial planning, loss of independence	Encourage pre-planning for funeral and other end of life decisions. Offer resources for other commitments e.g., caring for children and elderly parents. Encourage life review Encourage creation of legacy for children, grandchildren etc Encourage conversations regarding advance directives. Provide education on dying process. Provide support and education for sexual intimacy, if faced with physical limitations. Assess and explore spiritual and cultural beliefs and needs.

6. Transition care is now commonplace to support young people transferring from child to adult palliative care services. It has been identified that young adults require tailored services to meet their needs.
7. Adults can feel the increasing burdens of responsibility at their developmental stage and related pressures can impact their acceptance of their condition. At this time, the disease burden may also be higher and a need for greater medical interventions can be required to ease suffering.
8. There is acceptance in the literature that spiritual needs can influence an array of psycho-social needs. However, there remains an unease amongst health and social care professionals in beginning spiritual conversations and addressing spiritual needs. This points to a greater need for training in spiritual care and competences across professional boundaries.

Box 2.2 Reflective questions

1. Can you reflect on your age and developmental needs, how and in what ways do you think your life may be disrupted if a close family member was to be diagnosed with a serious illness?
2. Would you be comfortable in addressing others spiritual concerns? Would the age or developmental stage of the person impact on your readiness to support them?

References

Alvarez, E., Keegan, T., Johnston, E., et al., 2017. Adolescent and young adult oncology patients: disparities in access to specialised cancer centers. *Cancer, 123*(13), pp. 2516–2523.

Anbeek, C., 2017. World-viewing Dialogues on Preecarious Life: The Urgency of a New Existential, Spiritual, and Ethical Language in the Search for Meaning in Vulnerable life. *Essays in the Philosophy of Humanism, 25*(2), pp.171–185.

Balaguer, A., Martín-Ancel, A., Ortigoza-Escobar, D., Escribano, J., Argemi, J. 2012. The model of palliative care in the perinatal setting: a review of the literature. *BMC Pediatr 12*, p. 25. DOI: 10.1186/1471-2431-12-25

Bandeali, S., des Ordons, A.R. and Sinnarajah, A., 2020. Comparing the physical, psychological, social, and spiritual needs of patients with non-cancer and cancer diagnoses in a tertiary palliative care setting. *Palliative & Supportive Care, 18*(5), pp.513–518.

Bidegain, M. and Younge, N. 2015. Comfort care vs palliative care: is there a difference in neonates? *NeoReviews, 16*(6), pp.e333–e339.

Blakemore, S.J. and Choudhury, S. 2006. Development of the adolescent brain: implications for executive function and social cognition. *Journal of Child Psychology and Psychiatry*, 47(3-4), pp.296–312.

Bluebond-Langner, M. 1978. *The Private Worlds of Dying Children*. Princeton University Press.

Clark, J.K. and Fasciano, K., 2015. Young adult palliative care: Challenges and opportunities. *American Journal of Hospice and Palliative Medicine®, 32*(1), pp.101–111.

Damen, A., Exline, J., Pargament, K., Yao, Y., Chochinov, H., Emanuel, L., Handzo, G., Wilkie, D.J. and Fitchett, G., 2021. Prevalence, predictors and correlates of religious and spiritual struggles in palliative cancer patients. *Journal of Pain and Symptom Management, 62*(3), pp.e139–e147.

DeCourcey, D.D., Silverman, M., Oladunjoye, A. and Wolfe, J., 2019. Advance care planning and parent-reported end-of-life outcomes in children, adolescents, and young adults with complex chronic conditions. *Critical Care Medicine, 47*(1), pp.101–108.

Donoho, K., Fossa, M., Dabagh, S., Caliboso, M., Lotstein, D. and Nair, S., 2021. Compassionate extubation protocol to improve team communication and support in the neonatal intensive care unit. *Journal of Perinatology, 41*(9), pp.2355–2362.

Erikson, E.H., 1968. Identity and identity diffusion. Ch. Gordon and KJ Gergen (Eds.), *The Self in Social Interaction. Vol. I: Classic and Contemporary Perspectives,* New York (John Wiley & Sons) 1968, pp. 197–206.

Foulkes, L. and Blakemore, S.J., 2018. Studying individual differences in human adolescent brain development. *Nature Neuroscience*, *21*(3), pp.315–323.

Fraser, L.K., Gibson-Smith, D., Jarvis, S., Norman, P. and Parslow, R.C., 2021. Estimating the current and future prevalence of life-limiting conditions in children in England. *Palliative Medicine*, *35*(9), pp.1641–1651.

Graetz, D., Fasciano, K., Rodriguez-Galindo, C., Block, S.D., Mack, J.W. 2019. Things that matter: adolescent and young adult patients' priorities during cancer care. *Pediatr Blood Cancer*, *66*(9): e27883.

Hain, R., Devins, M., Hastings, R. and Noyes, J., 2013. Paediatric palliative care: development and pilot study of a 'Directory' of life-limiting conditions. *BMC Palliative Care*, *12*(1), pp.1–5.

Hinrichs, K.L., Woolverton, C.B. and Meyerson, J.L., 2022. Help me understand: providing palliative care to individuals with serious mental illness. *American Journal of Hospice and Palliative Medicine*, *39*(2), pp.250–257.

Huynh, L. and Moore, J., 2021. Palliative and end-of-life care for the older adult with cancer. *Current Opinion in Supportive and Palliative Care*, *15*(1), pp.23–28.

Jacobs, S., Perez, J., Cheng, Y., Sill, A., Wang, J., Lyon, M. 2014. Adolescent end of life preferences and congruence with their parents' preferences: results of a survey of adolescents with cancer. *Pediatr Blood Cancer*, *62*(4), pp.710–714.

Kirk, S. and Fraser, C., 2014. Hospice support and the transition to adult services and adulthood for young people with life-limiting conditions and their families: a qualitative study. *Palliative Medicine*, *28*(4), pp.342–352.

Knighting, K., Bray, L., Downing, J., Kirkcaldy, A.J., Mitchell, T.K., O'Brien, M.R., Pilkington, M. and Jack, B.A., 2018. Meeting the needs of young adults with life-limiting conditions: A UK survey of current provision and future challenges for hospices. *Journal of Advanced Nursing*, *74*(8), pp.1888-1898.

Levine, D.R., Mandrell, B.N., Sykes, A., Pritchard, M., Gibson, D., Symons, H.J., Wendler, D. and Baker, J.N., 2017. Patients' and parents' needs, attitudes, and perceptions about early palliative care integration in pediatric oncology. *JAMA Oncology*, *3*(9), pp.1214–1220.

Mallon, B., 2018. *Building Continuing Bonds for Grieving and Bereaved Children: A Guide for Counsellors and Practitioners*. Jessica Kingsley Publishers.

Mennito, S.H. and Clark, J.K., 2010. Transition medicine: a review of current theory and practice. *Southern Medical Journal*, *103*(4), pp.339–342.

Mitchell, S., Morris, A., Bennett, K., Sajid, L. and Dale, J., 2017. Specialist paediatric palliative care services: what are the benefits? *Archives of Disease in Childhood*, *102*(10), pp.923–929.

Needle, J.S., 2010. Home extubation by a pediatric critical care team: Providing a compassionate death outside the pediatric intensive care unit. *Pediatric Critical Care Medicine*, *11*(3), pp.401–403.

Office of National Statistics (2022) www.ons.gov.uk/peoplepopulationandcommunity/birthsdeathsandmarriages/deaths/bulletins/childhoodinfantandperinatalmortalityinenglandandwales/2020 (accessed 11 April 2022).

Perales, M.A., Drake, E.K., Pemmaraju, N., Wood, W.A. 2016. Social media and the adolescent and young adult (AYA) patient with cancer. *Curr Hematol Malig Rep*. 11(6), pp.449–455.

Reith, M. and Payne, M., 2009. *Social work in end-of-life and palliative care* (p. 29). Bristol: Policy Press.

Roeland, E., Lindley, L., Gilbertson-White, S., et al. 2019. End-of-life care among adolescent and young adult patients with cancer living in poverty. *Cancer, 126*(4), pp.886–893.
Rosen, D.S., Blum, R.W., Britto, M., et al. 2003. Society for Adolescent Medicine. Transition to adult health care for adolescents and young adults with chronic conditions: position paper of the Society for Adolescent Medicine. *J Adolesc Health*, 33, pp.309–311.
Sansom-Daly, U., Wakefield, C., Patterson, P., et al. End-of-life communication needs for adolescents and young adults with cancer: recommendations for research and practice. *J Adolesc Young Adult Oncol*, *9*(2), pp.157–165.
Sinclair, S., and Chochinov, H.M. (2012). Communicating with patients about existential and spiritual issues: SACR-D work. *Progress in Palliative Care*, *20*(2), pp.72–78.
Stilwell, P., Bhatt, A., Mehta, K., Carter, B., Bisset, M., Soanes, L. and Shankar, A., 2020. Preferred place of death in paediatric, teenage and young adult haemato-oncology patients: a retrospective review. *BMJ Supportive & Palliative Care*, *12*(e5), pp.e650–e653.
Sue, K., Mazzotta, P. and Grier, E., 2019. Palliative care for patients with communication and cognitive difficulties. *Canadian Family Physician*, *65*(Suppl 1), pp.S19–S24.
Together for Short Lives, 2017. *A neonatal pathway for babies with palliative care needs*. Together for Short Lives.
Together for Short Lives, 2017. A Perinatal Pathway for Babies with Palliative Care Need. Together for Short Lives.
Widger, K., Davies, D., Rapoport, A., Vadeboncoeur, C., Liben, S., Sarpal, A., Stenekes, S., Cyr, C., Daoust, L., Grégoire, M.C. and Robertson, M., 2016. Pediatric palliative care in Canada in 2012: A cross-sectional descriptive study. *Canadian Medical Association Open Access Journal*, *4*(4), pp.E562–E568.
Wiener, L., Weaver, M.S., Bell, C.J. and Sansom-Daly, U.M., 2015. Threading the cloak: palliative care education for care providers of adolescents and young adults with cancer. *Clinical Oncology in Adolescents and Young Adults*, *5*, p.1.
Zebrack, B.J., Block, R., Hayes-Lattin, B., Embry, L., Aguilar, C., Meeske, K.A., Li, Y., Butler, M. and Cole, S., 2013. Psychosocial service use and unmet need among recently diagnosed adolescent and young adult cancer patients. *Cancer, 119*(1), pp.201–214.

3 Caring relationships in children and young people's palliative care

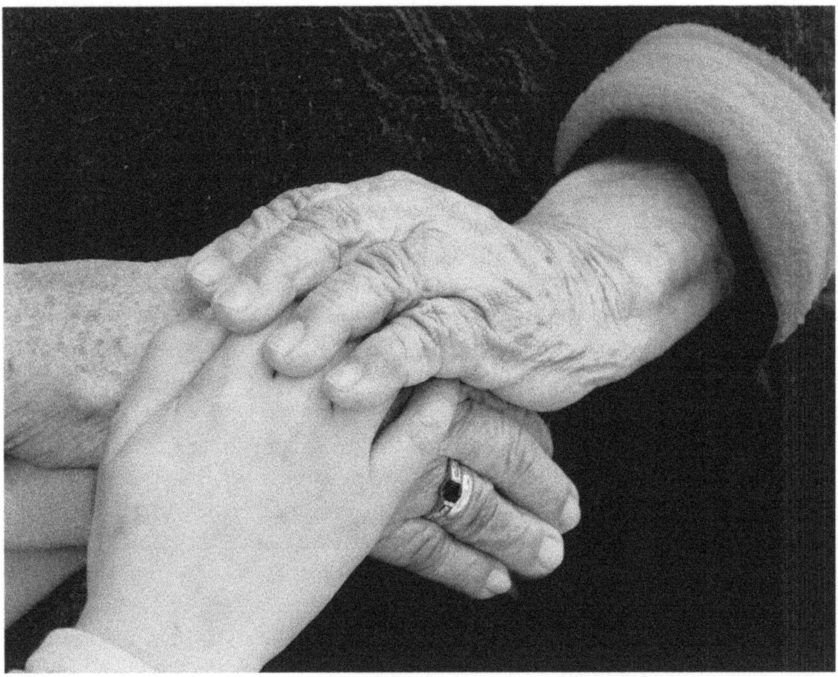

Figure 3.1 A photograph of multiple hands (of varied sizes/ages) entwined. Sourced from Google images.

Introduction

Children and young person's palliative care focuses much of its attention on individual-reported outcomes and individual and family centred care delivery. However, if we look beyond service delivery, we can explore the relational care needs of individuals. Empathy, compassion and mutuality are constructs relevant

DOI: 10.4324/9781003340287-4

to this discussion and are addressed in this chapter. Each can have positive effects on care experiences and allow individuals and families to feel that they are heard and that their views and experiences are both valued and validated.

Palliative care is relational, full of expectations around purpose and roles. Individuals can feel both comforted and empowered if there is a sense of mutuality in the cares provided. As such, 'Caring' involves 'being there' and 'being present' for individuals and families. Ideally, caring relationships exude trust, a meeting of needs, effective communication and a balance transfer of knowledge, energy and time (Buber, 1958).

Heidegger progresses our thinking delineating inauthentic and authentic caring. He suggested that 'Being-in-the-world' is made evident by appreciating that to Be is to care. Indeed, psychology regards caring as a quality we develop through our childhoods and constitutes a set of attitudes and behaviours mirrored by the nurturance of our parents (Erikson, 1968).

Person and family centred care

Person centred care or person centredness is emphasised in policy directives. The shift from medical paternalism to a more individual needs approach is welcomed. However, there remains in practice some diversity as to the willingness of professionals to embrace the individual with serious illness/their family taking on leadership in cares and them laying to one side their professional assertiveness to action in the wait for individual preferences to be asserted. All professionals want the best outcomes for individuals in their care, it takes experience and skill to hone down what is right and important for them, and we can only begin to appreciate this if we avail ourselves with the time and the patience to listen to the voices of children, young people and their families.

Since its inception children and young person's palliative care has been uniquely driven by a dual focus of individual and family centredness, the rhetoric has been strong. However, the models derived to assist professionals in their pursuits have not been totally effective, meaning there is continued scope to develop ways of working with families as it is appreciated especially that within palliative care, most often the unit of care is not just the individual with serious illness but also their family.

The family may be blood tied or not. The family is a group of individuals who share backgrounds and a willingness to support each other now and in future times (Boss and Dahl, 2014). These are the people who are providing hands on care, usually accompanying children and young people to appointments, who are in their presence at visits or being talked about in consultations. Throughout the time whereby the child or young person requires palliative care, families will also need support.

There are a few instances however, whereby professionals need to be more acutely aware of individual and family support needs.

Mosher et al. (2016) identified four challenges that affect all individuals with serious illness and their families:

1. Emotionally adjusting to the end stages of the condition
2. Managing all the demands of caregiving – the physical and the psychosocial.
3. Managing the uncertainty; and
4. Managing the suffering.

While all families have informational and support needs, there are instances that necessitate closer or more extensive family centred care provision, as highlighted by Park et al. (2018):

1. Where the family contains dependent children. These children will need support and preparation for loss. The single parent is of additional concern.
2. The family of a dying child – also raising other children and having to manage the related multitude of pressures. Siblings will need support to cope with the illness and death of their brother or sister. We know that a bereavement of this nature can be profound with long term effects. They also need support to cope with the parental attention that is focused away from them. Parents will need support to divide their attentions and to manage the emotional and physical burden of care and anticipatory grief.
3. Dysfunctional families, where there exists major communication breakdowns and relational conflicts. The burden of serious illness itself can break up relationships.
4. Families with high needs, where there are more than one loss, comorbid mental illness, trauma, homelessness and material disadvantages. Where needed, the palliative care teams may need to engage support of other services.

Empathy, sympathy, and compassion

An essential feature of person/family centred care has been the ability to appreciate other perspectives and to prioritise such over biomedical knowledge. This care moves us toward trying to understand better the holistic needs of the child or young person in living with their condition and their experience of the situation they are in. In supporting individuals and families, we feel a level of concern for them. When we feel concern then we are engaging in empathy. Empathy has been equated to having concern for the suffering, or where we understand the feelings of the other experiencing that suffering and where we feel we can respond to that suffering appropriately.

Two types of empathy have been delineated in the literature:

1. Cognitive empathy – a detached acknowledgment and understanding of an upsetting event/experience based on a sense of duty, and
2. Affective empathy – an acknowledgment and understanding of a person's situation by 'feeling with' the person (Lishner et al., 2011; Woolrych et al., 2020).

The term 'compassion' means to 'suffer with' and has been dictionary defined as 'a deep awareness of the suffering of another coupled with the wish to relieve it'. Compassion differs from sympathy (a none engaging feeling sorry) and empathy in that it is a behavioural approach, it involves actions taken to lessen the suffering in the observed. Gilbert and Choden (2013) discuss the connections that exist between empathy, sympathy and compassion. They conceptualise sympathy as an emotional reaction that does not engage the observer in feeling or thought. Empathy is more complex, requiring awareness, intuition and sometimes distress. Distress can result as the observer struggles with a need to make things right, to remedy the situation. Distress can also be a negative by product of the felt empathy. Whereas compassion forces the gaze away from the needs and activities of the self and efforts are more on operationalising support to promote the wellbeing of the other. Compassion, therefore, recognises suffering, relates to that suffering and responds to it instrumentally (Way and Tracy, 2012).

Over the last twenty five years, the concept of compassion has received much attention, both in public debate and health care discourse. The American philosopher Martha Nussbaum extensively explored compassion in her seminal discussion of the intelligence of emotions (Nussbaum, 2001). In situating her writing in an Aristotelian view of suffering and considering what suffering evokes, it is argued that compassion itself originates from the idea of 'the eudemonistic argument'. We are aware that as human beings we are vulnerable and subject to fate, what affects us and what we hold compassion for, could also one day affect us. In recognising our human vulnerability, we appreciate compassion.

Armstrong (2011), a British literary scientist, claimed compassion to equate to a type of consistent altruism, observable by engaging with 'the golden rule', which is to treat others as you yourself would like to be treated.

Compassion is also found to be a process of both intuition and explorative communication. Van der Cingel (2011) suggested that compassion contains the following attributes:

1. Attentiveness, to show an interest in others during a person-to-person encounter. Attentiveness is a conscious approach of showing interest or concern in or of another one person who shows interest in whatever issue is important for the other person. It also involves listening to the other and the listening can also evoke more telling or a greater conveying of the issue.
2. Involves silences and questioning, this allows the telling and shows interest in the telling.
3. Dialogue that then ensues can label and frame the suffering. The labelling act is also an act of acknowledgment. This is important, it makes it visible and stakes it out as meaningful or valuable, highlights it as something that should be known by others. Often the suffering needs to be confronted so that suffering can be supported. Professionals become experienced in recognising the nonverbal emotions such as grief, anger, fear and shame non-verbally, alongside inquiring about them.
4. When suffering is both verbalised and emotions shared the professional can be exposed to feeling and it is then that a mutuality is established. The

emotion becomes a shared emotion that is entrusted into the care of the professional.

5. Helping appreciates the needs of the individual. Nurses for example, often constitute compassion as their compulsion to help and to do.
6. The sixth attribute involves being present. To 'be there' requires physical and emotional presence. It also involves a conscious choice on part of the observer to be alert and notice what is necessary.
7. The last attribute encompasses understanding of suffering and the related emotionality.

These seven attributes of compassion can also be conceptualised as a process of grieving with.

Compassion and palliative care

Compassion is intrinsic to the care and support of those in need of palliative care. However, more recently authors have queried if this quality of palliative care continues to prevail. There is a new interest in the nature and place of compassion for palliative care globally. Compassion is a concept available to the self but one that holds better understanding across palliative care communities (Abel, 2018; Kellehear, 2012).

The Foucauldian concept 'care of the self' is important for us to appreciate prior to us being able to provide compassion for others. We need to care for ourselves before we have the capacity to care for others. Indeed, *'The care of the self is ethically prior, in that the relationship with oneself is ontologically prior'* (Foucault, 2003, p.30). This is broadly discussed in the health care literature and is beginning to surface in the palliative care discourse. Vachon et al. (2015) suggest a relationship exists between self-care and self-compassion and that self-compassion is a requirement to then have compassion for others. There is a need for further research on this as there remains a dearth of studies that have explored the inter relationship in palliative care because the ethos has always been to support the other who is the individual with serious illness and their family in need.

Self-care is defined as '*the self-initiated behaviour that people choose to incorporate to promote good health and general well-being*' (Sherman, 2004, p.52). Within health and social care, self-care is also aligned with self-resilience. A lack of self-care is therefore associated with compassion fatigue and professional burnout. As an ethical need, the *Oxford Textbook of Palliative Social Work* has described self-care as an element of best practice in palliative care (Altilio et al 2022).

Self-care

Self-care is a health promoting behaviour. However, the palliative care literature to date has transformed the concept into one of coping with stress and preventing burnout and fatigue. Managing stress is important but self-care means much more than that. If we are effectively providing ourselves with self-care, then we are hopefully at risk of much fewer negative impacts of stress in the first place.

A self-identity as a caring person is fundamental for those wanting professional caring roles. Especially within children and young person's palliative care whereby the culture is focused upon psychosocial support and the emotional needs of individuals and families. Roles within this area of health care are driven by the ability to be empathic and sensitive. This work also demands a professional emotional distance to be able to maintain professional identity and for self-preservation.

Emotional control is a widespread and accepted requirement of palliative care practice.

However, rather than the term emotional control, the term emotional labour may better help us to appreciate the lifeworlds of palliative care professionals. Emotional labour is a process that helps professionals balance the needs of the self, other and the demands of professionalism in health care. Both the emotion and emotional labour of health care is not acknowledged because it can be invisible in paid work, not least because it can be a role expectation (Brighton et al., 2019; Gray and Smith, 2009). Although there is acknowledgment of the interpersonal nature of care dominant work, and how working with repeated cases of grief, sadness and hopelessness involved with the care of the dying can take their effect. Few authors have made any connections to the concept of emotional labour in the palliative care literature. Yet, within broader health care, death is viewed as an 'emotional labour-inducing event' (Mann, 2005). Is this because professionals working in palliative settings are expected to be more resilient? They are more experienced in the care of the dying, so they need less support?

The concept of emotional labour extends beyond its existence in care relationships, to what is expected and what is normalised in palliative care. An understanding of such can help us to appreciate the role identities of professionals in this field of practice. Indeed the involved processes of emotional management *'can result in the inauthenticity of emotion and the alienation of self from self'* (Theodosius, 2012, p. 65).

Studies have historically explored how professionals cope and how they operationalise more attuned emotion focused coping strategies. For example, Skilbeck and Payne (2003) explored how nurse specialists cope with grief-related distress through different styles of emotional containment. Other studies have identified that coping with grief on the part of the professional is dictated by the broader cultural discourse. For example, death itself can be viewed as a *'merciful escape from suffering'* (Black and Rubinstein, 2005). In these instances, some professionals may begin to close themselves down emotionally by slowly detaching themselves in the later stages of an individuals illness. We all cope differently, and this can transfer to our professional practice. How we cope with the human condition and its finitude can provide an insight into the dynamics of emotional labour and the potential multiple identities of the self.

The narratives of participants in a study conducted by Funk et al. (2017) illustrate the complex and sometimes conflicting interpretations of the perceived acceptedness of expressed emotion in the workplace. Collaborating with individuals at the end of their lives is emotionally difficult and participants said they needed time and space, sometimes at work, sometimes at home, to be able to manage their grief related emotions. The needs of organisations, individuals and families served as barriers to their natural grief responses. Many participants suggested that their employees advocated to try and focus on the fact that they do or have done their best for the individuals in their care. In addition, their self-stigma of displaying grief publicly also predicated grief expression at work. Although some participants said they had tried to maintain an emotional distance from the individuals in their care, they also felt that such was impractical, and it also hindered their empathic, compassionate and direct cares for individuals and families which are essential to their role.

The work involved in palliative care involves a balancing of empathic caring and emotional distancing (Candrian, 2014). This can be most difficult at points of major transition be it from active to palliative care or from palliative to end of life care. The permitted professional norms of emotional distancing and internal grief suppression maintain a clinical containment of palliative care and a sanitised and routinised medicalisation of death. One is left to question how promoting this emotionally cleansed nature of caring is of long-term benefit to individuals, families and professionals. Further research is required to explore these realities and complexities in children and young people's palliative care.

Mutuality in care

It is commonly understood that, within nursing practice especially, exchanges of care can be both mutual and therapeutic. When the exchange is mutual it is perceived as compassionate. Hildegard Peplau (1952) originally identified this occurrence and encouraged the exploration of nursing as a relational practice. The philosophy of a mutual exchange forms the basis of modern-day service user involvement initiatives. The exchange between professionals, individuals and families in these contexts can be of mutual benefit. However, Barker and Buchanan-Barker (2004) have argued that the beneficial mutuality complicit in nursing practice has for many years been disregarded as influential to healing and psychosocial care. They advocated the 'Tidal model' to express the benefits of collaborative working. This 'joint journeying' through the individuals 'world of experience' can mean that kindness meets kindness, and opinions meet opinions, and we can increasingly bear witness to the other and get a sense of impacts, interests, and intentions. Aristotle would argue that mutuality is itself a form of reciprocity. Mutuality and mutual benevolence to this end are united.

Reciprocity and mutuality are often united in writings found in both the health care and social theory literature. It is therefore of use to palliative care practice to examine the concept and benefits of mutuality irrespective of how such can be influenced by the demands of social and institutional contexts.

The concept of mutuality holds value against social capital. Social capital and mutuality enable individuals to reach power and status that relationships without mutual support can be devoid of. Understanding social capital helps us to make sense of power relationships and how such can assist us in achieving mutuality. Mutuality is also shaped by the social frameworks that support presence and relations. Mutuality can allow the cultivation or development of egalitarian relationships and through mutuality we can also empower individuals to support others. Chan et al. (2022) further highlight the importance of mutuality and how encouraging processes of finding social commonalities, immersing oneself in family routines, supporting and enabling the wishes of those with serous illness and their families and engaging with individual's emotions enables health and social care professionals to achieve an interactive and relational understanding of individual and family needs. Such involvement and openness can also assist with broader compassionate community development as power differentials and related barriers are perceived to be reduced.

Empathic communication

Communication within palliative care is critical to caring relationships. Mutuality and compassion are both fostered via good empathic communication. Lowey (2008) identified that the qualities of a 'good' professional individual relationship included descriptions of trust, continuity of care and understanding. Effective communication is found to support advance care planning and can especially support those with verbal communication or capacity issues and in the instances of extremely sick or incredibly young children, can support parental and family decision making (Anderson et al., 2019).

Once a mutuality of care is achieved, palliative care professionals are more equipped to engage in empathic communication (Dahlin, 2015). For example, nurses can then hope to bridge the divide that can exist between the scientific information provided by physicians and the individual and family making care decisions. To this end health and social care professionals can ensure that with any decision made the individuals' values are upheld. The communication that occurs amongst professionals, individuals and families is an ingredient of quality care. Where open communication is maintained throughout the individual's illness trajectory, wellbeing can also be maintained and especially where decisions can be collaborative.

Milberg et al. (2012) reviewed experiences of palliative home care. Where care was perceived as good it was with open and empathic communication, encouraged by a team approach that valued individual experience. Other studies have noted that the effective and empathic communication of professionals enable family coping. Continuity of care out of hours is also appreciated (Hudson et al., 2019; Noble et al., 2015; Mehta et al., 2014).

Can we learn to be compassionate?

Through caring relationships health and social care professionals, individuals and families get to know each other and begin to appreciate the nuances of each other's personalities. For mutuality of care there is a need to appreciate each other's world views, the differences inherent can be at least initially explained by role in context but also age, social and gender disparities. But also, rapport must be built and time to transcend for the self to be shown to others. Where compassion is inherent in encounters and exchanges there is already a grounding of equality. It is the downplaying of any power differential that can encourage openness and a voicing of needs, expectations and emotion (Sawyer et al., 2021; Uitterhoeve et al., 2010).

Health and social care professionals have suggested the re is much worth in role models in practice and that it is the supporting of another's needs that encourages students to join the caring professions. There is continued debate as to whether those entering health and social care professional careers should be able to naturally be compassionate or if this is something that can be or is needed to be learnt. Many professionals in health and social care contexts use their knowledge from their engagement with and experiences of specific cases to grow in their practice. They become able to recognise individual cues because of the behavioural patterns they have seen before. With time they begin to appreciate what responses individuals may desire and if they want help. It is hard to determine if this knowledge of knowing what to do and when, is affected by the frequency of attending to individuals or because they are consciously using empathic communication skills. Regardless, the experiences of health and social care professionals interacting with individuals can be shared with students and analysed to explore good practice.

What can aide students in caring, is a development of their reflective skills. The reflexive professional can analyse their own actions in different contexts and its through being conscious of previous errors, distractions, or imperfections in our practices that we can expose the gaps in our compassionate ways of being towards individuals and families, be they related to being over or under emotional or just missing opportunities for dialogue (Adam and Taylor, 2014). Using the narratives of individuals, families and professionals has proven useful for qualified professionals and students to explore practice and to reflect upon emotions (Valen et al., 2019; van der Cingel, 2014). Sharing stories in a supportive environment with colleagues can also evoke an understanding of different interpretations and practices to achieve the same ends.

Social media and relationships with self and others

So far, the exploration of caring relationships has been focused on face-to-face transactions and with individuals that have a physical presence in our life worlds. However, increasingly in both contemporary practice and research we need to be mindful that we are now living in a technological age. Many of us use social media and this does not exclude children and young people with serious illness and their families. Indeed, social media can generate caring relationships as well as hinder them.

The internet and in particular social media platforms such as Facebook, Twitter, Instagram, TikTok and YouTube are relevant to everyone in resource rich countries and increasingly their use is minimalising the need for face-to-face communication. No longer do topics relative to illness, degeneration, death and dying have no outlet. Every day we can view and be part of live discussions or commentaries about such topics, via social media. If children and young people are living through a lack of knowledge or the mutual pretense created by family or professionals, it is quite possible that they can be enlightened about their own condition and prognosis through social media observances and interactions. And as such there is a void in the practice evidence base that allows us to accommodate for such.

Social media has had a significant impact on how those in palliative care and end of life live through their conditions and prepare for their deaths. Increasingly online communication is also likely to impact on how health and social care professionals are educated about individuals' wellbeing and wishes and how best to collaborate with them through their difficult transitions.

The dangers of social media are reported by the UK's General Medical Council and the British Medical Association, who have gone as far as issuing statements of caution. However, the debating on social media sites that occurs day in day out is intensifying, connecting individuals with others, and making the worlds of children and young people with serious illness and their families less lonely and unique.

In some cultures, there remains a need to be private about health status and being towards death. There has however been a noted increase in blogging and vlogging sites where both individuals with serious illness and professionals can be found to be documenting their experiences. In doing so, the taboo nature of such talk is being eliminated. Increasingly, health and social care professionals are holding a presence on sites such as Twitter and it is becoming commonplace to share knowledge from professional conferences on social media, meaning the public can access so much more previously hidden material. As an example, typing #eapc into the social media platform Twitter search engine will provide feedback from the most recent European Association for Palliative Care conference attendees and organisers. Such can be illuminating and counterbalance the non-scientific advice individuals and families can retrieve from general internet searches.

Increasingly researchers are capitalising on social media as a research tool and are also exploring how individuals cope by having access to and using social media platforms.

The nature of social media and end-of-life care and communication is explored in depth by Bassett (2015) and Sofka (2018) who argue that culturally, individuals from resource rich countries always try to accommodate modern day advances in how best to prepare for death and dying. Social media has become a new trend in that preparation. Social media use transcends to online death and dying ritual and can have impact on funerals, grief and memorialisation, inheritance and even archaeology.

This explosion of using digitalised social media has significantly increased in the last five years and is potentially of as much potential importance as the printing press invention of the fifteenth century (Aries). The practices of creating online illness and identity related material, private blogging or vlogging spaces and socially accessible diaries could be taking us forward into a quite different communicative, relational and caring world. A world whereby there is still much to learn and research to be done to expose both the benefits and pitfalls of social media and digital communication and to look at how best this increasing everyday practice and world development can be harnessed in children and young people's palliative care.

Chapter summary

Caring relationships in children and young people's palliative care involve much emotionality and sharing. Empathy, compassion, and mutuality although each difficult to define are incumbent in health and social care professional and individual and family care exchanges. Although deemed to some extent vocational, with good intentions, these qualities can be nurtured as it is through experience that professionals can become more accustomed to act with ease in mutual exchange with individuals and families. Care is not without emotional labour, and supervision can be needed to help professionals and students alike to reflect upon and manage the emotionality of their work. Technological advancements are changing the shape of relationships in palliative care. It is the role of children and young people's palliative care to maintain a mindfulness of individual and family needs and to move with the times, being involved in social media dialogue, and being prepared to support individuals and families who are impacted by what is shared by others.

Key issues

1. The ethos and practice of children and young people's palliative care is one of individual and family centredness.
2. Empathy, compassion, and mutuality of care are integral to good palliative care relationships with individuals and families.
3. Compassion is multifaceted and likened to being a grief-sharing endeavour.
4. Self-care is paramount to enable compassionate practice. For some this involves emotional distancing.
5. Palliative care relationships are evolving. The digital world is encouraging of digital online communication.
6. Social media identities and exchanges are participated in by health and social care professionals, individuals and families. Peer and informational support in children and young people's palliative care is therefore taking a new direction.

Box 3.1 Reflective questions

1. Do you think compassion can be taught?
2. Do you think it appropriate to maintain emotional distance from individuals and families? (How does this impact on caring relationships?)
3. How does social media impact on practices of social support provision and on other aspects of palliative care such as truth telling?

References

Abel, J., 2018. Compassionate communities and end-of-life care. *Clinical Medicine, 18*(1), p.6.

Adam, D. and Taylor, R., 2014. Compassionate care: Empowering students through nurse education. *Nurse Education Today, 34*(9), pp.1242–1245.

Altilio, T., Otis-Green, S. Cagle, J.G. (eds.), 2022. *Oxford Textbook of Palliative Social Work* (2nd Ed). Oxford University Press.

Anderson, R.J., Bloch, S., Armstrong, M., Stone, P.C. and Low, J.T., 2019. Communication between healthcare professionals and relatives of patients approaching the end-of-life: A systematic review of qualitative evidence. *Palliative Medicine, 33*(8), pp.926–941.

Armstrong, K., 2011. *Twelve steps to a compassionate life*. Random House.

Barker, P.J. and Buchanan-Barker, P., 2004. *The Tidal Model: A Guide for Mental Health Professionals*. Routledge.

Bassett, D.J., 2015. Who wants to live forever? Living, dying, and grieving in our digital society. *Social Sciences, 4*(4), pp.1127–1139.

Black, H.K. and Rubinstein, R.L., 2005. Direct care workers' response to dying and death in the nursing home: A case study. *The Journals of Gerontology Series B: Psychological Sciences and Social Sciences, 60*(1), pp. S3–S10.

Boss, P., and Dahl, C., 2014. Family therapy for the unresolved grief of ambiguous loss. In Kissane, D., Parnes, F. (Eds.), *Bereavement Care for Families*, pp. 171–182. Routledge.

Brighton, L.J., Selman, L.E., Bristowe, K., Edwards, B., Koffman, J. and Evans, C.J., 2019. Emotional labour in palliative and end-of-life care communication: A qualitative study with generalist palliative care providers. *Patient Education and Counseling, 102*(3), pp.494–502.

Buber, M. (1958). *I and Thou* (R.G. Smith, Trans.) (p. 11). Scribner.

Candrian, C., 2014. Taming death and the consequences of discourse. *Human Relations, 67*(1), pp.53–69.

Chan, W.S., Funk, L. and Thompson, G., 2022. A social capital perspective on social-medical collaboration in community end-of-life care in Hong Kong. *OMEGA-Journal of Death and Dying*, 0(0). https://doi.org/10.1177/00302228211066678

Codier, E., Muneno, L. and Freitas, E., 2011. Emotional intelligence abilities in oncology and palliative care. *Journal of Hospice and Palliative Nursing, 13*(3), pp.183–188.

Dahlin, C., 2015, November. Palliative care: Delivering comprehensive oncology nursing care. In *Seminars in Oncology Nursing* (Vol. 31, No. 4, pp. 327–337). WB Saunders.

Erikson, E.H., 1968. Identity and identity diffusion. *Ch. Gordon and KJ Gergen (Eds.), The Self in Social Interaction. Vol. I: Classic and Contemporary Perspectives,* 1968, pp. 197–206. John Wiley and Sons.

Foucault, M. 2003. *'Society Must Be Defended': Lectures at the Collège de France, 1975–1976*, D. Macey et al., trans. Picador.

Froggatt, K., 1998. The place of metaphor and language in exploring nurses' emotional work. *Journal of Advanced Nursing*, *28*(2), pp.332–338.

Funk, L.M., Peters, S. and Roger, K.S., 2017. The emotional labour of personal grief in palliative care: Balancing caring and professional identities. *Qualitative Health Research*, *27*(14), pp.2211–2221.

Gilbert, P., and Choden, E. 2013. *Mindfulness Compassion*. Robinson.

Gray, B. and Smith, P., 2009. Emotional labour and the clinical settings of nursing care: the perspectives of nurses in East London. *Nurse Education in Practice*, *9*(4), pp.253–261.

Hudson, B.F., Best, S., Stone, P. and Noble, T.B., 2019. Impact of informational and relational continuity for people with palliative care needs: a mixed methods rapid review. *BMJ Open*, *9*(5), p.e027323.

Kellehear, A., 2012. *Compassionate Cities*. Routledge.

Lishner, D.A., Batson, C.D. and Huss, E., 2011. Tenderness and sympathy: Distinct empathic emotions elicited by different forms of need. *Personality and Social Psychology Bulletin*, *37*(5), pp.614–625.

Lowey, S.E., 2008. Letting go before a death: A concept analysis. *Journal of Advanced Nursing*, *63*(2), pp.208–215.

Mann, S., 2005. A health-care model of emotional labour: An evaluation of the literature and development of a model. *Journal of Health Organization and Management*, *19*(4/5), pp.304–317.

Mehta, A., Chan, L.S. and Cohen, S.R., 2014. Flying blind: sources of distress for family caregivers of palliative cancer patients managing pain at home. *Journal of Psychosocial Oncology*, *32*(1), pp.94–111.

Milberg, A., Wåhlberg, R., Jakobsson, M., Olsson, E.C., Olsson, M. and Friedrichsen, M., 2012. What is a 'secure base' when death is approaching? A study applying attachment theory to adult patients' and family members' experiences of palliative home care. *Psycho-Oncology*, *21*(8), pp.886–895.

Mosher, C.E., Winger, J.G., Given, B.A., Helft, P.R. and O'Neil, B.H., 2016. Mental health outcomes during colorectal cancer survivorship: a review of the literature. *Psycho-Oncology*, *25*(11), pp.1261–1270.

Noble, H., Price, J.E. and Porter, S., 2015. The challenge to health professionals when carers resist truth telling at the end of life: a qualitative secondary analysis. *Journal of Clinical Nursing*, *24*(7–8), pp.927–936.

Nussbaum, M.C., 2001. *The Fragility of Goodness: Luck and Ethics in Greek Tragedy and Philosophy*. Cambridge University Press.

Park, M., Lee, M., Jeong, H., Jeong, M. and Go, Y., 2018. Patient-and family-centered care interventions for improving the quality of health care: A review of systematic reviews. *International Journal of Nursing Studies*, *87*, pp.69–83.

Peplau, H.E., 1952. The psychiatric nurses' family group. *The American Journal of Nursing*, *52*(12), pp.1475–1477.

Rodriguez, A. and King, N., 2014. Sharing the care: the key-working experiences of professionals and the parents of life-limited children. *International Journal of Palliative Nursing*, *20*(4), pp.165–171.

Sawyer, J.M., Higgs, P., Porter, J.D. and Sampson, E.L., 2021. New public health approaches to palliative care, a brave new horizon or an impractical ideal? An integrative literature review with thematic synthesis. *Palliative Care and Social Practice, 15*, p.26323524211032984.

Sherman, D.W., 2004. Nurses' Stress & Burnout: How to care for yourself when caring for patients and their families experiencing life-threatening illness. *AJN The American Journal of Nursing, 104*(5), pp.48–56.

Skilbeck, J. and Payne, S., 2003. Emotional support and the role of clinical nurse specialists in palliative care. *Journal of Advanced Nursing, 43*(5), pp.521–530.

Sofka, C., 2018. Adolescents' use of social media and digital technology to cope with life-threatening illness and loss: what parents and supportive adults should know. *ChiPPS E-Journal Pediatric Palliative and Hospice Care, 53*, p.18.

Theodosius, C. (2012). 'Feeling a feeling' in emotion management. In Spencer, D., Walby, K., Hunt, A. (Eds.), *Emotions Matter: A Relational Approach to Emotions*, pp. 63–85. University of Toronto Press.

Uitterhoeve, R.J., Bensing, J.M., Grol, R.P., Demulder, P.H.M. and Van Achterberg, T., 2010. The effect of communication skills training on patient outcomes in cancer care: a systematic review of the literature. *European Journal of Cancer Care, 19*, pp. 442–457.

Vachon, B., Désorcy, B., Gaboury, I., Camirand, M., Rodrigue, J., Quesnel, L., Guimond, C., Labelle, M., Huynh, A.T. and Grimshaw, J., 2015. Combining administrative data feedback, reflection and action planning to engage primary care professionals in quality improvement: qualitative assessment of short term program outcomes. *BMC Health Services Research, 15*(1), pp.1–8.

van der Cingel, M., 2011. Compassion in care: A qualitative study of older people with a chronic disease and nurses. *Nursing Ethics, 18*(5), pp.672–685.

van der Cingel, M., 2014. Compassion: The missing link in quality of care. *Nurse Education Today, 34*(9), pp.1253–1257.

Valen, K., Holm, A.L., Jensen, K.T. and Grov, E.K., 2019. Nursing students' perception on transferring experiences in palliative care simulation to practice. *Nurse Education Today, 77*, pp.53–58.

Way, D., and Tracy, S.J., 2012. Conceptualizing compassion as recognizing, relating and (re) acting: A qualitative study of compassionate communication at hospice. *Communication Monographs, 79*(3), pp. 292–315.

Woolrych, T., Eady, M.J. and Green, C.A., 2020. Authentic empathy: A cultural basis for the development of empathy in children. *Journal of Humanistic Psychology*, early online publication, June 19, 2020. https://doi.org/10.1177/0022167820934222

4 The perceived vulnerabilities of children and young people with serious illness

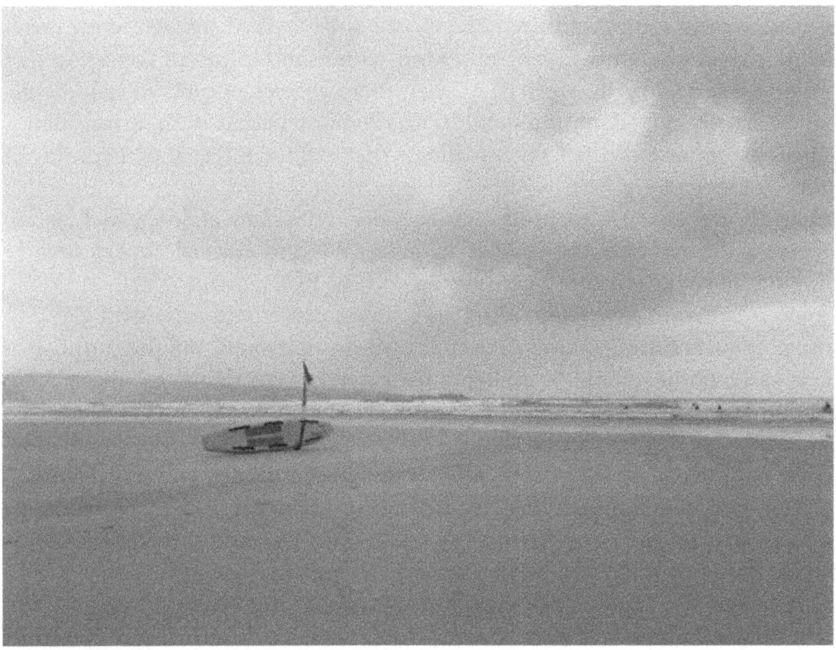

Figure 4.1 Photograph of a desolate beach.
Photograph taken by Alison Rodriguez.

Introduction

There has been a lot of literature published that suggests that disabled people are marginalised, infantilised and perceived as asexual (see Earl and Blackburn, 2020). This perception of vulnerability is because of the assumption that individuals with serious illness are more vulnerable to abuse and harm. There exists a social stigma about children and young people with serious illness,

DOI: 10.4324/9781003340287-5

and how they need protection from the details of their condition and possible futures because of their vulnerability. Children and young people with serious illness are viewed as individuals with different needs to children and young people without serious illness. These stigmatised views can influence poor mental health outcomes for children and young people with serious illness who want to belong and integrate into society irrespective of their physical health needs. Notwithstanding these issues of discriminatory gaze, children and young people are subject to symptoms and periods of poor health and degeneration that require supportive cares to enable them to function socially and to have their voices heard. With increasing frailty children and young people may struggle to maintain control, and suffer psychological impacts resultant of body image concerns, the trauma of physical health care interventions, the social upset of not being able to establish friendships or romantic relationships and their emotional and physical struggle with issues such as pain management, sleep problems, nausea and impaired cognition due to illness and treatment impacts. As such there are perceptions of vulnerabilities externally placed upon on children and young people with serious illness and issues because of their serious illness that induce internal perceptions of vulnerability too.

Health and social care professionals, working within children and young people's palliative care, are present in individual and familial experiences of suffering and will at times bear witness to fear, loss, sadness, anger, and guilt. Children and young people with serious illness can emotionally struggle with their physical suffering, burden, loneliness, meaninglessness, and the purpose of their being. Some may indicate freely their need to communicate about these matters, others may require a little encouragement. There is however a current appreciation of how exploring these issues and their related emotions with individuals, and where appropriate families, can be both needed and therapeutic.

'Knowing' and 'not knowing' can influence well-being and relationships. To protect the child or young person from 'knowing' can feed the professional or familial desire to lower the burden or even to enhance the individual's quality of life across the trajectory of their condition that they have left to live. The desire to protect the child or young person feeds the external perception of these individuals being vulnerable and different and evolves from the privileged position of others 'knowing'. To 'know' can lead to over protectiveness and barrier building. From the perspective of the child or young person with serious illness, their unwillingness to further burden their significant others can also lead to critical issues not being broached. They are aware of how upsetting their situation is for family and carers and they can internalise their needs so as not to cause further stress for others.

Perceptions around vulnerabilities due to age and norms relative to cultural heritage can also impact on both the willingness and comfort a family member or professional has in sharing or withholding information about a child or young person's illness and their prognosis and in discussing their age and developmentally appropriate needs.

Truth telling

In many resource rich countries, truth telling is an expected norm in exchanges of health and social care and related advice. This can be conceived as the current ethical position. Historically however, there was more focus upon paternalism and beneficence. It is only since the beginning of the twentieth century that we have developed a respect for 'patient' autonomy. To this end, if a health or social care professional fails to be honest with individuals in their care, then they deny these individuals their right to autonomy. If an individual is armed with an understanding (developmentally appropriate) of the nature of their condition, their potential illness trajectories, and treatment options, then they can have some level of mastery over their wellbeing.

Is honesty always the best policy?

Ones cultural heritage dictates to a large degree an individual's views and beliefs. Culture shapes our meaning making and how we may cope with suffering and living towards dying, our decision making and whether we want to hear bad news and what our end-of-life wishes may be. In the UK, a great deal of emphasis is placed upon individual autonomy, informed consent and truth telling. However, these norms and values can be at conflict with some residents of the population. Those with different heritage may place greater value on family involvement and decision making over autonomy for example (Clark and Phillips, 2010). This is congruent with the focus upon beneficence in some cultures over autonomy. Where beneficence is a priority then concealment of truths is advocated to maintain hope and emotional wellbeing (Kagawa-Singer and Blackhall, 2001).

Western countries generally promote the autonomy dominant paradigm of health care. As such, open communication and a degree of sadness is expected, not least so any future fears can be established and relieved. This approach to health and social care means that individuals (mostly adults) with serious illness are encouraged to have open conversations about advanced planning and end of life wishes. In all cultures there is an acceptance of the fact that truthful communication between professionals and individuals has benefits. However, disagreement exists regarding the degree of any benefit that can ensue from open discussion of a life shortening prognosis (Shahidi, 2010).

Collusion (where family members request withholding information from the individual with serious illness) is often found in communities that hold more value on family over individual decision making. Several studies have highlighted how such family preferences are threaded within communities throughout the world, including Asia, Africa, Europe, and the Middle East (Beyraghi et al., 2011; Khalil, 2013). However, it is common for health care professionals in the west to care for families with alternative values (Chittem and Butow, 2015). Ethical conflicts can particularly affect the delivery of end-of-life care. However, literature is available that considers how best to respond to families who are at conflict with western health care norms. Guidelines advocate that individual autonomy is not a priority in some cultures and advocate that cultural values are relevant to person centred care. We therefore need to be open to alternative perspectives, not least to be empathetic and to promote compassion. If we do not acknowledge that different values exist, then the quality of palliative care is compromised.

Autonomy is a right, not an obligation, and so, if we force decision making or truth telling on individuals and families uncomfortable with such practices, then this is a violation of their integrity. Therefore, health and social care professionals working in children and young people's palliative care benefit from training in difficult communication scenarios. If we are so focused on individual autonomy and rights we may fail to hear and respect family values and so we are then at risk of conducting our practices with a cultural bias (Blackhall et al., 1995; Kaihlanen et al., 2019).

These real-world practice conflicts are recognised in UK palliative and end-of-life care policy (Sleeman et al., 2021) and the Mental Capacity Act (2005), where family involvement is recognised (with the individual's consent). The resuscitation guidance by the General Medical Council (General Medical Council. Treatment and Care Towards the End of Life (2023)) also advocate the inclusion of individual and family in discussions but note that medical decisions are those to be made by physicians.

Plato wrote about 'merciful lies', he recognised their value in supporting hope and although he argued that we should all be truth telling beings, he acknowledged that there would be times whereby physicians could be forgiven of their need to lie (Fan and Li, 2004). Holding back the truth can be ethically challenging for health and social care professionals. It can be difficult for them to act if there appears to be conflict between individual and family desires and it can be difficult to follow familial tradition if this restricts autonomy. Concealment of the truth for many can feel disrespectful. However, Beyene (1992) suggested that individuals themselves are the most able to judge their own health severity. We are also now able to independently access much information related to symptoms and diagnoses/prognoses on-line that can impact knowledge status (Kynoch et al., 2019).

Not all cultures however, are preoccupied with preparing for death. For individual's affiliated with the Islamic faith, only God permits death. With knowledge of dying, we may give up on life and this is not congruent with the religious teachings and so a loss of faith in God can result. Therefore, to openly discuss the prospect of dying and its probable time frame with an individual of staunch islamic faith, would be deemed as disrespectful to both the individual and their religion. To this end, health and social care professionals can also be influenced by their own belief systems and can have difficulty with truth telling norms. The ETHICUS (End-of-Life Practices in European Intensive Care Units) study discovered that physicians from southern Europe were highly protective of individuals in their care and as such were found to communicate little about life shortening prognoses to either individuals or families (Sprung et al., 2007). Hartog et al. (2022) completed a follow up study to explore if there had been any changes in prognostic communication over a 16-year period across European Intensive Care Units. It was highlighted that end-of-life decisions are being increasingly discussed but there remains communication practice differences across regions, with a north south divide still evident. In addition, patient preferences with respect to their end of life communication were not commonly known, with physicians only aware of the end of life wishes of 20% of their patients.

Individuals with serious illness, especially children and young people, are reliant on the health and social care team to support their best interests as they enter palliative and end of life care. The cultural values of health and social care professionals influence the immediacy of truth telling in negotiation with families. It is agreed however, that the interests of the child or young person should dominate over the values of the treating or supporting health and social care professionals. It is also acknowledged that many children and young people with palliative care needs are bodily aware and can sense their failing health and so will have sometimes already have contemplated bad news before it is communicated. A diagnosis that infers a shortened life expectancy prognosis is upsetting but can be what both the individual and their family are expecting. Of course, there will be children and young people with life limiting conditions from birth, but if they have cognitive awareness, will encounter and display extreme upset or disbelief in entering a phase of degeneration. There will also still be individuals who have had no prior inclination and for those, the disclosure can be more traumatic (Stein et al., 2019; Voltz et al., 1998).

Cultural preferences

Living in multicultural societies we embrace diversity and divergent cultural practices. Cultural relativism however, with respect to our ethical standards in health and social care poses challenges. If truth telling practices should override others, this can be deemed both prejudicial and insensitive. Many cultures advocate value systems that they believe prioritise family and community welfare and as such there exists an argument that western bioethical norms represent minority thinking. In many Asian cultures, illness is accepted to be a family event and not just an individual concern (Searight and Gafford, 2005). The family is an immediate support system; therefore, autonomy cannot hold the same meaning because family is central to all decisions and actions. Studies confirm that in Middle Eastern communities, families want to protect individuals from bad news (Silbermann and Hassan, 2011). A Japanese study of family behaviours in palliative care described how the family has a protective role in shielding the patient from a painful diagnosis (Surbone, 2008). Physicians in the east respect the autonomy of the family unit (Chattopadhyay and Simon, 2008; Yamaguchi et al., 2021).

However, like any advocated cultural norm there is always a degree of diversity. A comprehensive literature review that explored the views of individuals from Egypt, Iran, Israel and Palestine, Jordan, Lebanon, Kuwait, Pakistan, Saudi Arabia, Turkey, and the United Arab Emirates, highlighted the variability of truth telling beliefs and practices (Bou Khalil, 2013). For example, 52% of Pakistani residents said they would desire full prognosis disclosure (Ishaque et al., 2010). Whereas the same response was higher amongst Turkish respondents 88%, with 92% suggesting it was the treating physician's responsibility to deliver bad news. Israeli studies have also discovered that physician practices are variable. With 61% of subspecialists and 25% of family practitioners claiming to always disclose to individuals. In Kuwait however, 67% of physicians supported full disclosure practices with the same percentage in Pakistan arguing for none disclosure, suggesting that disclosure causes unnecessary psychological distress (Ben Natan et al., 2009). In addition, cancer disclosures were reported as cruel (Aljubran, 2010). Indeed, a number of studies have found a relationship between prognostic disclosure, psychological distress, and psychopathology and reduced quality of life (Hui et al., 2021; Wiener et al., 2012).

With these cultural differences in mind, it is easier to see how individuals from diverse backgrounds may find it challenging to talk to health and social care professionals about treatment and care options. Furthermore, language difficulties may further hinder challenging conversations.

Breaking bad news

Talking to loved ones about important end-of-life decisions can spark a complicated land mine of emotions. So much so, many people put it off until it is too late and there are many instances both in the media and the literature that cite difficulties and inadequacies in bad news disclosure. Sometimes it is not the detail of the information that is the trigger for poor disclosure outcomes, but the nature of its delivery. Breaking bad news is a real communication challenge for all health and social care professionals. This is an event whereby the quality of the health or social care professional's communication skills are exposed to potential self-detriment.

What do we mean by bad news?

Several definitions exist with respect to what we mean by bad news. Ptacek and Eberhadt (1996) suggested that bad news is where a medical situation involves no hope and the lifestyle of the individual will be affected, or there is a situation that will threaten psychological and/or physical wellbeing. Ultimately, bad news is conceptualised as such when the felt response of the individual involves a decline in cognitive, behavioural or emotional wellbeing and those deficits continue following the communication exchange. Alternatively, Buckman (1984) stated bad news massively changes future worldviews in a negative way. Following an in-depth narrative analysis of 138 individuals' written accounts detailing their experience of being told they had cancer, Salander (2002) suggested that bad news is more than an event, it is a process that also involves the individual reflecting on the expertise of treating physicians and how well or not they have protected them from dangers. A frequently operationalised definition of bad news, however, is that which is communicated that includes bad, sad or significant detail which negatively transforms the individuals' expectations and perceptions for their present and future (Fallowfield and Jenkins, 2004). This definition takes the understanding away from bad news just being about diagnosis, prognosis or treatment and can relate to several life events or events on the medical pathway and it involves feelings relative to the now and the future.

The definition by Fallowfield and Jenkins (2004) also emphasises the fact that what determines issues as 'bad news' is the perception itself of the news, as classified by the person receiving it. We all have the capacity to interpret news in diverse ways. How we interpret the information can be influenced by a number of factors, including our expectations, values, life experiences and social connectedness. This is notwithstanding the fact that most people will find the disclosure of a shortened life to be difficult but for other issues it is not always easy to forecast how the news will be taken. However, if we can appreciate there will be a subjective difference in how individuals and families will react, the disclosure event can be less pressured for professionals (Eggly et al., 2006).

In summary, we classify news as bad in a health and social care context where the information given will change the recipients' view of their future in a negative way. The negative weight of the news can be determined by the individuals' understanding of their situation leading up to the news disclosure; the less they know, the greater the negative impact (Buckman, 2005).

There are, however, also differences in expectations regarding the amount of information desired by individuals and about what aspects of care/treatment/ the condition (Cain et al., 2018). For example, some individuals may want the focus of talk to be on intervention options and intentions for support, whereas others may just want to know the relevant statistics relating to longevity (Innes and Payne, 2009). Regardless, most individuals in receipt of bad news just want to know as soon as possible and to have trust in what is conveyed (Cleary et al., 2010).

Why is breaking bad news important?

Laying cultural preferences aside, working within the individual autonomy framework, studies have repeatedly shown that most individuals desire to be fully informed about their condition and its expected trajectory. When they are kept updated, it is felt that there is an increasing confidence in health care relationships, and this provides individuals with an ongoing confidence to ask questions about their status. If individuals and families have full news disclosure, then they can plan for their futures because they can manage their predicament in realistic terms. Indeed, health care professionals suggest when they participate in the process of breaking bad news, they subsequently have stronger and more effectual relationships with individuals with serious illness and their families (Miller et al., 2022; Warnock et al., 2010).

There are, however, always situations when it is not considered useful to disclose information. Some individuals do not desire total facts as it would hinder their ways of coping. Cultural differences have already been identified. Therefore, it is always important to ascertain individual preferences about information disclosure and sharing. It is also important to note that although individuals may indicate a preference for no information disclosure, as their condition progresses and they experience bodily changes, then they may reach a point of wanting to be told.

Why is breaking bad news difficult?

The individual's right to be told about the full extent of their condition and impact on their longevity has been bound in law in some resource rich countries (Bousquet et al., 2015). However, in practice there are still instances where news will not be given or will be slightly distorted for many reasons, by health and social care professionals. Professionals need to balance legal requirements with not wanting to cause burden and manage individual and family wishes (Sarafis et al. 2014).

There can be a truth telling hesitance for several reasons. Truth telling is emotionally difficult for all and the reactions of individuals and families cannot always be predicted. Individuals can express anger, tears, hysteria, denial, verbal abuse, threatening behaviour, bargaining and silence (Campbell et al., 2010). With knowledge of the literature and experience of having had previous distressing reactions, it is understandable that health and social care professionals will be concerned about not just how to deliver the bad news but how it will be received.

Managing the responses requires effective communication skills and time, which is not always do-able in more hectic health care settings (Fallowfield and Jenkins, 2004). Health and social care professionals can also struggle with guilt because they have been unable to 'fix things' even though nothing could ever be achieved given the circumstances. The providers of bad news also have a lot of their own issues to manage in the context of the discussion. Not knowing what the best way is to say what they need to say, waiting on the right moment and being unsure if they have answered any questions effectively causes great worry and can induce a professional reluctance to disclose. A further reason for hesitance can be the knowledge that hope can be diminished. This is of major concern when the news relates to prognoses and end of life care. Unlike discussions about a change in health state or ability, a life shortening prognosis holds incredible weight.

Studies that have explored individuals' experiences of receiving bad news reveals the detail of subsequent difficulties in maintaining hope (Millet et al., 2022). Therefore, professional hesitance for this reason is not unfounded. However, the same body of evidence suggests that the provision of truthful information does not mean that all sense of hope will be diminished, it is an opportunity to reframe that hope, looking toward the future, quality of life and what yet can be achieved in life. Campbell et al. (2010) investigated how best to balance realism and hope and states:

> *When we worry about destroying hope we are generally referring to a very specific hope of getting better or living longer. But hope is a complex, multidimensional and*

> *above all flexible construct... One can shift from hoping for a cure... to hoping to go home from the hospital. Such a shift in the things one hopes for requires a reframing of goals to meet the realities at hand... [a reality] that none of us would wish for.* (p.461)

Bad news does not always lessen hope, it can mean that new goals are created. With the gift of a given timeline, we can resolve life conflicts, mend relationships and express our wishes. Evidence around breaking bad news supports the premise again that it is not just the content of the news that matters but how it is delivered. Delivered sensitively and being responsive to individual and family questioning can help individuals and families to cope, to still see they have some life direction and purpose, some level of hope, but this requires skill, knowledge, and expertise.

Emotional labour

Being tasked with the role of breaking bad news involves much emotional labour. Emotional labour is defined as managing other people's feelings. A distinct element of emotional labour is emotional regulation. James (1989) states emotional labour facilitates and controls how emotion is expressed in social situations. Hochschild (1983/2012) and Smith (1992) argue that emotional labour is determined by three characteristics:

1. Involves voice-to-voice or face-to-face contact with a member of the public, i.e., the individual with serious illness or family.
2. The professional is expected to engage emotionally in the other, i.e. there is a likelihood of emotional upset.
3. The professional in their pursuit must be able to control their own emotionality.

Emotional labour is more commonplace within health care. Identifying the prevalence of emotional labour in health care allows for supportive strategies to be put in place, such as clinical supervision, training, and peer reflection. Emotional labour is itself categorised as a skill or area of expertise. However, this is difficult to conceptualise fully, and its efficacy is difficult to measure. Breaking bad news involves a lot of emotional labour and can explain why some professionals choose to refrain from that role.

Delivering bad news causes professional discomfort. Historically, distancing tactics were provided to assist professionals in their truth telling endeavours. Maguire (1985) highlighted cases of both nurses and physicians using distancing tactics for emotional protection. Such tactics included the use of closed questions, hinging on time constraints so the news could be delivered quickly, and a quick exit could ensue, moving quickly onto practical tasks to avoid subsequent questioning and for some professionals the worry was so great their distancing involved delaying on not providing the news at all. These tactics were not always conscious but on reflection could be deemed as self-protective behaviours. Dunniece and Slevin (2000) suggested that distancing tactics are also because professionals do not want to create more individual distress. Bloom et al. (2022) highlight how health and social care professionals worry about how to assess patient and caregiver understanding during and following prognostic disclosure.

Frameworks for breaking bad news

Because of the emotional labour involved in bad news delivery, a number of guiding frameworks have been created to support professionals. Although a number of local and national guidelines exist (that provide tips and protocol), professionals will often draw on the framework of Buckman's S.P.I.K.E.S (Setting, Perception, Information, Knowledge, Empathy and Summarising) strategy (2005). Buckman's strategy explores the emotional issues that need to be considered when delivering bad news and guides professionals in ways to remember important facts through the emotional context. Like other guidance documents there are limitations that reside with there being no clear instruction in how to bolster one's own confidence levels and in particular what communication skills need strengthening for effective delivery.

Fallowfield et al. (2002) explored the training of 160 doctors in 34 UK cancer centres and identified that bespoke training drastically improved baseline communication skills. A national programme for advanced communication skills training is now in place following the publication of the National Institute for Health and Clinical Excellence (NICE) guidance 'Improving Supportive and Palliative Care for Adults with Cancer' (2004). This is a three-day course and is offered to senior nurses, allied health professionals and physicians, employed in cancer and palliative care. Using problem-based learning the course is centred on participant needs. In most cancer and palliative care teams there is now a requirement that at least one member has completed this training.

Warnock et al. (2010) explored nurse's difficulties in delivering bad news. A number of interesting findings were derived, previously unremarked upon in the literature. Often it was difficult to ascertain what the individual already knew and indeed what they had already been told by other professionals. Unexpected deterioration also meant that news sometimes had to be delivered over the telephone, which meant the emotional response was more difficult to gauge. Synnot et al. (2018) explored health communication research priorities for those with serious illness. They suggested prioritising research that would explore structural barriers to health communication and that would help health and social care professionals develop their communication skills and strategies.

Prognostic disclosure to children

Prognostic disclosure to children has perpetually challenged health and social care professionals and parents. There was no research or tailored training on this matter until the 1950s (Mack et al., 2016). Therefore, professionals felt unprepared in their practice. When considering the discussion of prognosis with children it is important that we understand how the child will comprehend information. Initial texts on children's understandings of death were derived from the psychological literature. Nagy's seminal article of 1948 is cited widely in this literature. Based on qualitative research with children it was claimed that children less than nine years old were incapable of comprehending death, whereas those above nine could understand to the same degree as adults. However, children started presenting with more complex conditions and there appeared an increasing need for disclosure. Nagy's work was used to suggest young children would not have their prognosis disclosed because they would not be able to appreciate its meaning. Indeed, it was thought that they were unable to experience fear or anxiety of dying. Children were routinely excluded from prognosis discussions and often any consultation. For children above nine years the literature from the 1960s also promoted a nondisclosure approach.

A review of this literature details four main arguments against prognosis disclosure specifically to children with cancer (Mack and Joffe, 2014; Mack and Smith, 2012; Rosenberg et al., 2016).

1. There was a fear that there could be inaccuracies in diagnosis.
2. There was worry that such knowledge could cause unneeded distress and disclosure could result in suicide. Concealment would require creative reasoning however and often blatant lying.
3. Children rarely demand information. This lack of demand was interpreted as a lack of need whereas others saw it as a coping strategy.
4. Also, there was concern that disclosure could disrupt family relationships.

However, the early 1970s marked a tidal change in opinion and approach, with four arguments to be communicatively open with children:

1. First, it was realised that children are often already aware of their predicament. Binger et al. (1969) interviewed the parents of twenty-three deceased children. Fourteen parents stated they had withheld prognostic information from their child yet eleven of these parents thought their child knew without being told. John Spinetta, psychologist, was instrumental in bringing about this awareness of children possessing a knowingness. He argued children wanted to know for sure the reality of their illness (Wiener et al., 2012; Kao and Goh, 2013).
2. The effort required to conceal truths can be emotionally exhausting and lead to more difficult conversations and familial relationships when the child sometimes becomes aware of their reality (Rosenberg et al., 2017; Mack and Joffe, 2014)
3. When children guessed their prognosis because of their diagnosis it was pondered that children were not asking questions because they were afraid rather than they were uninterested (Kao and Goh, 2013).
4. Emerging research began to agree that open communication was of support to dying children (Wang et al., 2011).

In the following years, the evidence base grew. By the 1980s, the practice moved from do not tell to do tell. However, the prognosis disclosure situation is now being reconsidered. We now appreciate, not least from adult studies, that prognostic disclosure is complex, both for the disclosing professional and recipient. There are current debates around how and when we should disclose to children. We are no longer supportive of a do or do not tell philosophy. Instead, there is an understanding that we should consider disclosure on a nature of the case basis. There is also a contemporary awareness however, that because of the complex nature of disclosure and its psychosocial demands and outcomes, that professionals are becoming increasingly paternalistic and hesitant to break bad news.

Professional considerations

Age and developmental ability help professionals to estimate the child's understanding of their condition. However, the child's illness experiences are of greater relevance. In addition, children like adults may have preferences for disclosure or not. Research before the millennium centred on parental needs and preferences and few studies explored children's perceptions (Natan et al., 2009). However, it was noted that both parents and health and social care professionals could misinterpret child desires. More recent studies detail that most adolescents can interpret prognostic disclosure and prefer to be involved in end-of-life decision making (Bates and Kearney, 2015; Wiener et al., 2022).

A proportion of children will shy away from these conversations to protect their parents who they perceive to be already burdened by their condition. In these instances, some children may need private discussions away from parents to communicate their needs. It is also important to note that like adults, children's views on disclosure can alter through the course of their illnesses (Bluebond-Langner et al., 2010).

Health professionals therefore have the challenging task of working out what needs to be disclosed, to whom and at what point. To assist health and social care professionals, they can benefit from training to interpret both parental and child communication cues and to explore what communication styles are needed for the unique situations that can present themselves in child parent encounters (Wiener et al., 2013; Weiner et al., 2022). In addition, any communication with family in children and young people's palliative care is dictated by parents/guardians. Most parents/guardians want to be fully informed. However, some do not want their children to have full disclosure to protect their wellbeing. In these circumstances, health and social care professionals can adopt 'subtle diplomacy' whereby they become the central communicator, listening to both perspectives of parents and the child, trying to achieve a middle ground to ensure person and family centred care, and that all needs are met (Bluebond-Langner et al., 2010).

Supporting children and young people with serious illness to live life to the fullest

Research with children and young people with serious illness is impeded by several challenges. There can be limited access to participants and there can be difficulties for potential participants to engage in studies due to their symptom burden and ability to self-report. Still, wherever possible it is important to invite children and young people with serious illness to participate in research so that their voices can be heard and taken account of in practice developments and interventions. Namisango et al. (2019) undertook a systematic review of studies that have highlighted the symptomatic concerns of children and young people with serious illness. The review also provides suggestions for health and social care professional support to enable children and young people with serious illness to live fuller and happier lives (see Figure 4.2).

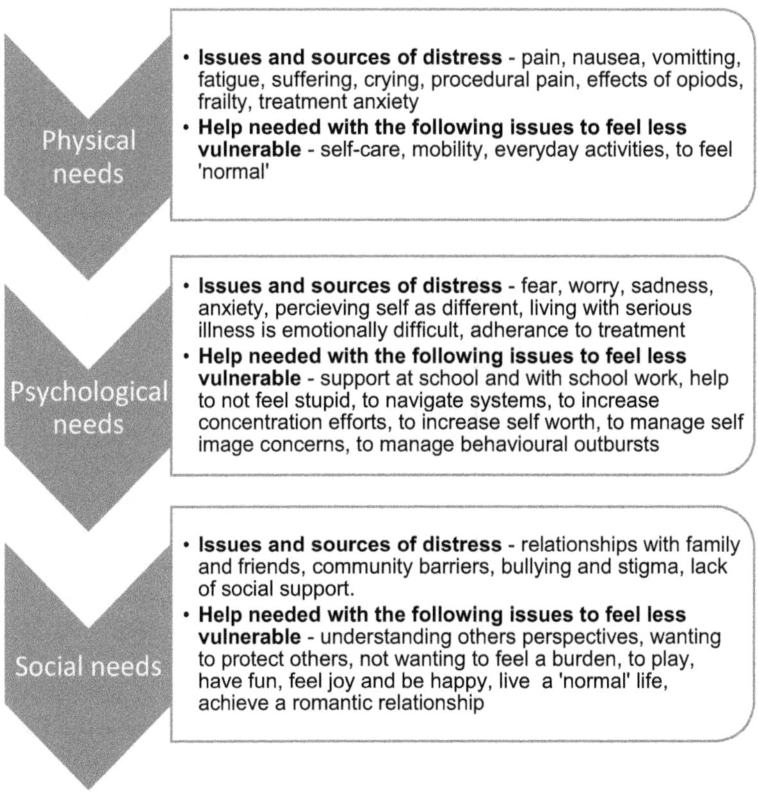

Figure 4.2 Children and young people's needs with serious illness.
Adapted from Namisango et al., 2019.

Studies in the review included an array of methodologies, some including self-report from the perspectives of young people with serious illness, others included observations and the views of parents and health and social care professionals. The findings are beneficial for us to try and understand perspectives on what it is like for children and young people to live with serious illness and experience associated vulnerabilities.

Supported decision making

Supported decision making can be actioned in diverse ways. Usually, it is needed when people with cognitive impairments need help with making decisions (Kohn et al., 2012). With serious illness and advancing disease can come increasing dependency, so trying to maintain a system of autonomous decision making for some individuals can become too difficult to achieve (Donchin, 2001). Adopting an approach to care that involves supported decision making engages professionals in further exploring the contexts of individuals' lives and their histories. This unveils more detailed pictures of the identities of individuals concerned and their individual needs and perceived vulnerabilities. This research work on behalf of professionals can help them to be more considerate of the child or young person when they or others need to consider with families, preferences for treatment, care, and support.

If supported decision making is actioned over advanced directives, then there can be increased wellbeing for the child or young person. This approach is not alien to all families. Some will routinely talk through and about decisions with their children (Wright, 2020).

Advanced care planning

Advanced care planning (ACP) conversations and goals of care (GoC) discussions are often written about in a similar vein in the literature. Each involves discussing with individuals their values and beliefs, and what concerns them the most about their situation and future. With this knowledge, health and social care professionals can aim to provide care that is aligned with the individual's personhood and choices. Advanced care planning for adults in the UK is now well established in palliative care practice and considered a factor within the Gold Standards Framework, the purpose of which is to achieve high-quality end of life care (Hughes et al., 2018).

Advanced care planning for children and adolescents is less developed. Although the Convention of Children's Rights (1989) recognises the right for children to be involved in medical decision making. Legislation and policy in the United Kingdom (such as The Children Act 2004 and the Mental Capacity Act 2005) allow decisions to be made by others for children assuming best interests and yet also promote the involvement of children and young people in their care decision making. The use of advanced care planning for children and young people is evident in the UK and has been increasingly operationalised since 2010, however not all those who could access this practice end up developing an advanced care plan. In fact, children and young people show similar uptake to figures seen internationally, where there is less motivation and support in children and young people's palliative care for advanced care planning (Kavalieratos et al., 2015).

There are a few tools that can help the shared decision-making process, including The Wishes Document (Fraser et al., 2010) and My Choices (Wiener et al., 2012) and approaches to care including Family Centred Advance Care Planning (Kimmel et al., 2015) that can encourage family units to follow the advanced care planning process. In addition, Together for Short Lives has developed resources to support children and young people's care planning and the use of these tools. In the last five years there has also been the launch of the Child and Young Person's Advance Care Plan; an informative website with documentation and access to training and allied information for different audiences about advanced care planning with children and young people (Child and Young Person's Advance Care Plan Collaboration, accessed 2022). Involving children and young people in their advanced care planning can improve their wellbeing, but to be effective, health and social care professionals need to have the experience and training to provide appropriate guidance and support.

Futile treatment

While health and social care professionals seek to accentuate and respect the individual's identity, they also seek to support their cultural needs. They can face many conflicts if families however insist on prolongation of active treatment or of the dying process. It can be difficult for professionals to support the decision making of families and their distress and balance their life prolongation wishes against professional knowledge of conditions and the limited resources of healthcare availability. When individuals or families desire futile treatment at the end of life, professionals do consider the sanctity of life in religions but will recommend not engaging in aggressive therapies that could also make the individuals end of life traumatic (Westra, 2009).

According to Islam, the physician must be able to prove that death is inevitable and if that cannot be achieved then everything should be done to maintain life (Surbone, 2008). However, the futility of end-of-life treatment is difficult to both be certain of and define. A number of factors come into play, including, the effect any treatment or intervention would have on quality and length of life, emotional costs, financial costs and success rates. It is therefore common that experience and value judgements will be drawn upon (Rodriguez and Young, 2006). Because of the level of uncertainty that can exist over the nature of some conditions, their impact and time frame, it has been identified that many Saudi Arabian physicians do not comment on their expectations regarding the utility or futility of available treatments and their will to disclose if they think individuals in their care are close to death (Younge et al., 1997).

Physicians practice within the boundaries of medical utility and futility, establishing the benefits and costs of treatment for everyone in their care. In the UK, the General Medical Council guidelines state that physicians are not ethically obligated to provide futile treatment (General Medical Council, 2023). Within the UK health care system decision making is very much based upon the futility and benefit of treatments/interventions. Although much attention is placed on helping individuals and families to understanding why something will be not actioned to extend or maintain life. In this respect ultimate decisions of this nature are not dictated by either individual or family. This could be quite opposite in areas of the world that fully embrace cultural beneficence. Health care professionals therefore do not inquire about permission to not treat or remove a treatment. Instead, they inform individuals and families as to what is happening and why. There is evidence to suggest that where end of life decisions are fully informative and collaborative that individuals have a better quality of life towards death, receive less futile interventions and are a lower cost to health care systems (Zhang *et al.*, 2009).

Chapter summary

In many areas of the world, the practices of truth telling are intrinsic to palliative care practices. Therefore, it can be difficult if there are families wanting to take the lead in decision making over individuals and indeed if there are desires to conceal truths by families from individuals. Several other factors can also impact on truth telling in families, including the complexities and uncertainties of conditions and the age of the individual. Without doubt hope can impact on wellbeing and there is fear that sometimes prognostic knowledge can impact negatively on quality of life.

We are in an age of rapid change with increasing global multiculturalism, and it is fair to say there are many diverse cultural and belief systems that need to be managed within the palliative care world. It can be challenging for professionals when faced with belief systems that are not necessarily congruent with mainstream practices or ethical norms. However, it is the professional's role to adapt where possible their practice to accommodate ethical models so that the needs of individuals and families from diverse cultural backgrounds can be met.

There are also difficulties faced when individuals and families feel like they do not want to 'give up'. Emotions can impact judgement, but it can be difficult for professionals to negotiate requests for futile treatment against condition realities and cultural needs. Professionals need guidance to communicate with children, young people and families going through these turbulent times. Guidelines and frameworks exist with respect to delivering bad news, and often experience and reflection can develop the efficacy of delivery. This role is not always relished, and so specific training has been implemented especially for those who work in children and young people's palliative care as they may not have addressed it in their core training.

The key to good palliative delivery for professionals is effective communication, access to advance skills training, a knowledge of how best to work with supportive or shared decision making and a knowledge of the social constructed notion of the individual as being vulnerable. Professionals can guide families to be more open and able to work with bad news and to not be frightened of the child or young person also having some form of awareness, even before they are told. Much growth in individual wellbeing and familial relationships can be observed if individuals can reflect on their lives lived and plan for their futures.

Key issues

1. Due to age and the nature of life limiting and threatening conditions, children and young people with serious illness are viewed as vulnerable. This view of vulnerability can lead to social stigmas.
2. In addition, the physical, psychological and social impacts of serious illness can lead to children and young people with serious illness feeling vulnerable.
3. In the UK and other resource rich countries in the west, there is a dominant practice of truth telling in palliative care. This is not always seen in some cultures where there can be a preference to conceal news and be totally reliant on family decision making. However, regardless of truth telling norms there can remain a protectiveness towards children and young people with serious illness leading to a hesitance to tell them full details of their condition.
4. Breaking bad news involves much emotional labour on the part of health and social care professionals and families.
5. There is specialist training and guidance now in place for those working in children and young people's palliative care, however, there remains hesitance on the part of some professionals to divulge bad news.
6. Truth concealment can also arise because of issues related not just to the individual's age but to the complexities of conditions.
7. There can be uncertainties regarding condition longevity and fears as to what impact the bad news could have on the emotional wellbeing of the child, young person, family and relationships.
8. Professionals need to cater their truth telling, support and interventions to the unique needs of each child, young person and family.

Reflective questions

1. Would you want to know all details of your illness prognosis if you were in receipt of palliative care? (Would there be limits?)
2. What aspects of serious illness and associated vulnerabilities do you perceive to be the most difficult?

3. What aspects of bad news delivery and the emotional labour of it, do you think could be delivered in core training? (Be mindful that child and young person palliative populations are growing, and the specialism is becoming more diverse).

References

Aljubran, A.H., 2010. The attitude towards disclosure of bad news to cancer patients in Saudi Arabia. *Annals of Saudi Medicine, 30*(2), pp.141–144.

Bates, A.T. and Kearney, J.A., 2015. Understanding death with limited experience in life: dying children's and adolescents' understanding of their own terminal illness and death. *Current Opinion in Supportive and Palliative Care, 9*(1), p.40.

Beyene, Y., 1992. Medical disclosure and refugees. Telling bad news to Ethiopian patients. *Western Journal Of Medicine, 157*(3), p.328.

Beyraghi, N., Mottaghipour, Y., Mehraban, A., Eslamian, E. and Esfahani, F., 2011. Disclosure of cancer information in Iran: a perspective of patients, family members, and health professionals. *Iranian Journal of Cancer Prevention, 4*(3), p.130.

Binger, C.M., Ablin, A.R., Feuerstein, R.C., Kushner, J.H., Zoger, S. and Mikkelsen, C., 1969. Childhood leukemia. *New England Journal of Medicine, 280*(8), pp.414–418.

Bluebond-Langner, M., Belasco, J.B. and Wander, M.D., 2010. 'I want to live, until I don't want to live anymore': involving children with life-threatening and life-shortening illnesses in decision making about care and treatment. *Nursing Clinics, 45*(3), pp.329–343.

Blackhall, L.J., Murphy, S.T., Frank, G., Michel, V. and Azen, S., 1995. Ethnicity and attitudes toward patient autonomy. *JAMA, 274*(10), pp.820–825.

Bloom, J.R., Marshall, D.C., Rodriguez-Russo, C., Martin, E., Jones, J.A. and Dharmarajan, K.V., 2022. Prognostic disclosure in oncology-current communication models: a scoping review. *BMJ Supportive & Palliative Care, 12*(2), pp.167–177.

Bousquet, G., Orri, M., Winterman, S., Brugière, C., Verneuil, L. and Revah-Levy, A., 2015. Breaking bad news in oncology: a metasynthesis. *Journal of Clinical Oncology, 33*(22), pp.2437–2443.

Buckman, R.A., 2005. Breaking bad news: the SPIKES strategy. *Community Oncology, 2*(2), pp.138–142.

Buckman, R., 1984. Breaking bad news: why is it still so difficult?. *British Medical Journal (Clinical Research ed.), 288*(6430), p.1597.

Cain, C.L., Surbone, A., Elk, R. and Kagawa-Singer, M., 2018. Culture and palliative care: preferences, communication, meaning, and mutual decision making. *Journal of Pain and Symptom Management, 55*(5), pp.1408–1419.

Campbell, T.C., Carey, E.C., Jackson, V.A., Saraiya, B., Yang, H.B., Back, A.L. and Arnold, R.M., 2010. Discussing prognosis: balancing hope and realism. *The Cancer Journal, 16*(5), pp.461–466.

Chattopadhyay, S. and Simon, A., 2008. East meets West: Cross-cultural perspective in end-of-life decision making from Indian and German viewpoints. *Medicine, Health Care and Philosophy, 11*(2), pp.165–174.

Child and Young Person's Advance Care Plan Collaboration. Child and Young Person's Advance Care Plan. http://cypacp.uk/ (accessed 20 May 2022).

Chittem, M. and Butow, P., 2015. Responding to family requests for nondisclosure: The impact of oncologists' cultural background. *Journal of Cancer Research and Therapeutics*, *11*(1), p.174.

Clark, K. and Phillips, J., 2010. End of life care: The importance of culture and ethnicity. *Australian Family Physician*, *39*(4), pp.210–213.

Cleary, M., Hunt, G.E., Escott, P. and Walter, G., 2010. Receiving difficult news: Views of patients in an inpatient setting. *Journal of Psychosocial Nursing and Mental Health Services*, *48*(6), pp.40–48.

Convention of Children's Rights, 1989. www.ohchr.org/en/instruments-mechanisms/instruments/convention-rights-child (accessed 10 May 2022).

Department of Health's End of Life Care Strategy: Promoting High Quality Care for All Adults at the End of Life. https://assets.publishing.service.gov.uk/government/uploads/system/uploads/attachment_data/file/136431/End_of_life_strategy.pdf (accessed 15 March 2022).

Dixon, J, Knapp, M., 2020. Learning from international models of advance care planning to inform evolving practice in England. NIHR. School for Social Care Research.

Donchin, A., 2001. Understanding autonomy relationally: toward a reconfiguration of bioethical principles. *The Journal of Medicine and Philosophy*, *26*(4), pp.365–386.

Dunniece, U. and Slevin, E., 2000. Nurses' experiences of being present with a patient receiving a diagnosis of cancer. *Journal of Advanced Nursing*, *32*(3), pp.611–618.

Eggly, S., Penner, L., Albrecht, T.L., Cline, R.J., Foster, T., Naughton, M., Peterson, A. and Ruckdeschel, J.C., 2006. Discussing bad news in the outpatient oncology clinic: rethinking current communication guidelines. *Journal of Clinical Oncology*, *24*(4), pp.716–719.

Fallowfield, L. and Jenkins, V., 2004. Communicating sad, bad, and difficult news in medicine. *The Lancet*, *363*(9405), pp.312–319.

Fallowfield, L.J., Jenkins, V.A. and Beveridge, H.A., 2002. Truth may hurt but deceit hurts more: communication in palliative care. *Palliative Medicine*, *16*(4), pp.297–303.

Fan, R. and Li, B., 2004. Truth telling in medicine: The Confucian view. *Journal of Medicine and Philosophy*, *29*(2), pp.179–193.

Fraser, J., Harris, N., Berringer, A.J., et al. 2010. Advanced care planning in children with life-limiting conditions – the wishes document. *Arch Dis Child*, 95, 79–78.

Ganzini, L., Goy, E.R., Miller, L.L., Harvath, T.A., Jackson, A. and Delorit, M.A., 2003. Nurses' experiences with hospice patients who refuse food and fluids to hasten death. *New England Journal of Medicine*, *349*(4), pp.359–365.

General Medical Council. 2023/2022. Treatment and Care Towards the End of Life: Good Practice in Decision-Making www.gmc-uk.org/ethical-guidance/ethical-guidance-for-doctors/treatment-and-care-towards-the-end-of-life (accessed 5 January 2023).

Gill, C.J., 2004. Depression in the context of disability and the 'right to die'. *Theoretical Medicine and Bioethics*, *25*(3), pp.171–198.

Hartog, C.S., Maia, P.A., Ricou, B., Danbury, C., Galarza, L., Schefold, J.C., Soreide, E., Bocci, M.G., Pohrt, A., Sprung, C.L. and Avidan, A., 2022. Changes in communication of end-of-life decisions in European ICUs from 1999 to 2016 (Ethicus-2)-a prospective observational study. *Journal of Critical Care*, *68*, pp.83–88.

Hayhoe, B, Howe, A, Gillick, M, et al., 2011. Advance care planning under the Mental Capacity Act 2005 in primary care. *Br J Gen Pract*, *61*, e537–e541.

Hochschild, A.R., 1983/2012. The managed heart. In *The Managed Heart*. University of California Press.

Hughes, B., O'Brien, M.R., Flynn, A. and Knighting, K., 2018. The engagement of young people in their own advance care planning process: a systematic narrative synthesis. *Palliative Medicine, 32*(7), pp.1147–1166.

Hui, D., Mo, L. and Paiva, C.E., 2021. The importance of prognostication: impact of prognostic predictions, disclosures, awareness, and acceptance on patient outcomes. *Current Treatment Options in Oncology, 22*(2), pp.1–14.

Innes, S. and Payne, S., 2009. Advanced cancer patients' prognostic information preferences: a review. *Palliative Medicine, 23*(1), pp.29–39.

Ishaque, S., Saleem, T., Khawaja, F.B. and Qidwai, W., 2010. Breaking bad news: exploring patient's perspective and expectations. *Journal of the Pakistan Medical Association, 60*(5), p.407.

James, N., 1989. Emotional labour: skill and work in the social regulation of feelings. *The Sociological Review, 37*(1), pp.15–42.

Jimenez, G, Tan, WS, Virk, AK, et al., 2018. Overview of systematic reviews of advance care planning: summary of evidence and global lessons. *J Pain Symptom Manag, 56*, pp. 436–459.e25.

Kagawa-Singer, M. and Blackhall, L.J., 2001. Negotiating cross-cultural issues at the end of life: You got to go where he lives. *JAMA, 286*(23), pp.2993–3001.

Kaihlanen, A.M., Hietapakka, L. and Heponiemi, T., 2019. Increasing cultural awareness: qualitative study of nurses' perceptions about cultural competence training. *BMC Nursing, 18*(1), pp.1–9.

Kao, Y.H. and Goh, C.R., 2013. The practice of nondisclosure of advanced cancer diagnosis in Singapore: a continuing challenge. *Singapore Med J, 54*(5), pp.255–258.

Kavalieratos, D., Ernecoff, N.C., Keim-Malpass, J. and Degenholtz, H.B., 2015. Knowledge, attitudes, and preferences of healthy young adults regarding advance care planning: a focus group study of university students in Pittsburgh, USA. *BMC Public Health, 15*(1), pp.1–7.

Khalil, R.B., 2013. Attitudes, beliefs and perceptions regarding truth disclosure of cancer-related information in the Middle East: a review. *Palliative & Supportive Care, 11*(1), pp.69–78.

Kimmel, A.L., Wang, J., Scott, R.K., et al. 2015. FAmily CEntered (FACE) advance care planning: study design and methods for a patient-centered communication and decision-making intervention for patients with HIV/AIDS and their surrogate decision-makers. *Contemp Clin Trials*, 43, pp. 172–178.

Kohn, N.A., Blumenthal, J.A. and Campbell, A.T., 2012. Supported decision-making: A viable alternative to guardianship. *Penn St. L. Rev., 117*, p.1111.

Kynoch, K., Ramis, M.A., Crowe, L., Cabilan, C.J. and McArdle, A., 2019. Information needs and information seeking behaviors of patients and families in acute healthcare settings: A scoping review. *JBI Evidence Synthesis, 17*(6), pp.1130–1153.

Longmore, P.K., 1995. Medical decision making and people with disabilities: A clash of cultures. *Journal of Law, Medicine & Ethics, 23*(1), pp.82–87.

Lund, S., Richardson, A., May, C., 2015. Barriers to advance care planning at the end of life: an explanatory systematic review of implementation studies. *PLoS One, 10*, e0116629

Mack, J.W., Cronin, A.M. and Kang, T.I., 2016. Decisional regret among parents of children with cancer. *Journal of Clinical Oncology, 34*(33), pp.4023–4029.

Mack, J.W. and Joffe, S., 2014. Communicating about prognosis: ethical responsibilities of pediatricians and parents. *Pediatrics*, *133*(Supplement_1), pp. S24–xS30.

Mack, J.W. and Smith, T.J., 2012. Reasons why physicians do not have discussions about poor prognosis, why it matters, and what can be improved. *Journal of Clinical Oncology*, *30*(22), pp.2715–2717.

Maguire, P., 1985. Barriers to psychological care of the dying. *Br Med J (Clin Res Ed)*, *291*(6510), pp.1711–1713.

Mental Capacity Act, 2005. www.legislation.gov.uk/ukpga/2005/9/contents (accessed 31 May 2022)

Miller, E.M., Porter, J.E. and Barbagallo, M.S., 2022. The experiences of health professionals, patients, and families with truth disclosure when breaking bad news in palliative care: A qualitative meta-synthesis. *Palliative & Supportive Care*, *20*(3), pp.433–444.

Myers, J., Cosby, R., Gzik, D., Harle, I., Harrold, D., Incardona, N. and Walton, T., 2018. Provider tools for advance care planning and goals of care discussions: a systematic review. *American Journal of Hospice and Palliative Medicine®*, *35*(8), pp.1123–1132.

Nagy, M. (1948). The child's theories concerning death. *Journal of Genetic Psychology*, *73*, 3–27.

Namisango, E., Bristowe, K., Allsop, M.J., Murtagh, F.E., Abas, M., Higginson, I.J., Downing, J. and Harding, R., 2019. Symptoms and concerns among children and young people with life-limiting and life-threatening conditions: a systematic review highlighting meaningful health outcomes. *The Patient-Patient-Centered Outcomes Research*, *12*(1), pp.15–55.

Natan, M.B., Shahar, I. and Garfinkel, D., 2009. Disclosing bad news to patients with life-threatening illness: differences in attitude between physicians and nurses in Israel. *International Journal of Palliative Nursing*, *15*(6), pp.276–281.

National Institute for Health and Clinical Excellence (NICE) guidance 'Improving Supportive and Palliative Care for Adults with Cancer' (2004). www.nice.org.uk/guidance/csg4 (accessed 11 April 2022)

Ptacek, J.T. and Eberhardt, T.L., 1996. Breaking bad news: a review of the literature. *JAMA*, *276*(6), pp.496–502.

Quill, T.E. and Brody, H., 1996. Physician recommendations and patient autonomy: finding a balance between physician power and patient choice. *Annals of Internal Medicine*, *125*(9), pp.763–769.

Rodriguez, K.L. and Young, A.J., 2006. Patients' and healthcare providers' understandings of life-sustaining treatment: are perceptions of goals shared or divergent? *Social Science & Medicine*, *62*(1), pp.125–133.

Rosenberg, A.R., Starks, H., Unguru, Y., Feudtner, C. and Diekema, D., 2017. Truth telling in the setting of cultural differences and incurable pediatric illness: a review. *JAMA Pediatrics*, *171*(11), pp.1113–1119.

Rosenberg, A.R., Wolfe, J., Wiener, L., Lyon, M. and Feudtner, C., 2016. Ethics, emotions, and the skills of talking about progressing disease with terminally ill adolescents: a review. *JAMA Pediatrics*, *170*(12), pp.1216–1223.

Sarafis, P., Tsounis, A., Malliarou, M. and Lahana, E., 2014. Disclosing the truth: a dilemma between instilling hope and respecting patient autonomy in everyday clinical practice. *Global Journal of Health Science*, *6*(2), p.128.

Searight, H.R. and Gafford, J., 2005. Cultural diversity at the end of life: issues and guidelines for family physicians. *American Family Physician*, *71*(3), pp.515–522.

Salander, P., 2002. Bad news from the patient's perspective: an analysis of the written narratives of newly diagnosed cancer patients. *Social Science & Medicine, 55*(5), pp.721–732.

Shahidi, J., 2010. Not telling the truth: circumstances leading to concealment of diagnosis and prognosis from cancer patients. *European Journal of Cancer Care, 19*(5), pp.589–593.

Silbermann, M. and Hassan, E.A., 2011. Cultural perspectives in cancer care: impact of Islamic traditions and practices in Middle Eastern countries. *Journal of Pediatric Hematology/Oncology, 33*, pp. S81–S86.

Sleeman, K.E., Timms, A., Gillam, J., Anderson, J.E., Harding, R., Sampson, E.L. and Evans, C.J., 2021. Priorities and opportunities for palliative and end of life care in United Kingdom health policies: a national documentary analysis. *BMC Palliative Care, 20*(1), pp.1–10.

Smith, P., 1992. *The Emotional Labour of Nursing: Its Impact on Interpersonal Relations, Management, and Educational Environment.* Macmillan International Higher Education.

Sprung, C.L., Maia, P., Bulow, H.H., Ricou, B., Armaganidis, A., Baras, M., Wennberg, E., Reinhart, K., Cohen, S.L., Fries, D.R. and Nakos, G., 2007. The importance of religious affiliation and culture on end-of-life decisions in European intensive care units. *Intensive Care Medicine, 33*(10), pp.1732–1739.

Stein, A., Dalton, L., Rapa, E., Bluebond-Langner, M., Hanington, L., Stein, K.F., Ziebland, S., Rochat, T., Harrop, E., Kelly, B. and Bland, R., 2019. Communication with children and adolescents about the diagnosis of their own life-threatening condition. *The Lancet, 393*(10176), pp.1150–1163.

Stein, G. L., and Kerwin, J. (2010). Disability perspectives on health care planning and decision-making. *Journal of Palliative Medicine, 13*(9), pp. 1059–1064.

Surbone, A., 2008. Cultural aspects of communication in cancer care. *Supportive Care in Cancer, 16*(3), pp.235–240.

Synnot, A., Bragge, P., Lowe, D., Nunn, J.S., O'Sullivan, M., Horvat, L., Tong, A., Kay, D., Ghersi, D., McDonald, S. and Poole, N., 2018. Research priorities in health communication and participation: international survey of consumers and other stakeholders. *BMJ Open, 8*(5), p.e019481.

The Children Act, 2004. www.legislation.gov.uk/ukpga/2004/31/contents (accessed 10 May 2022).

Voltz, R., Akabayashi, A., Reese, C., Ohi, G. and Sass, H.M., 1998. End-of-life decisions and advance directives in palliative care: a cross-cultural survey of patients and health-care professionals. *Journal of Pain and Symptom Management, 16*(3), pp.153–162.

Wang, D.C., Guo, C.B., Peng, X., Su, Y.J. and Chen, F., 2011. Is therapeutic non-disclosure still possible? A study on the awareness of cancer diagnosis in China. *Supportive Care in Cancer, 19*(8), pp.1191–1195.

Warnock, C., Tod, A., Foster, J. and Soreny, C., 2010. Breaking bad news in inpatient clinical settings: role of the nurse. *Journal of Advanced Nursing, 66*(7), pp.1543–1555.

Westra, A.E., Willems, D.L. and Smit, B.J., 2009. Communicating with Muslim parents: 'the four principles' are not as culturally neutral as suggested. *European Journal of Pediatrics, 168*(11), pp.1383–1387.

Wiener, L., Bedoya, S., Battles, H., Sender, L., Zabokrtsky, K., Donovan, K.A., Thompson, L.M., Di Ciccone, B.B.L., Babilonia, M.B., Fasciano, K. and Malinowski, P., 2022. Voicing their choices: advance care planning with adolescents and young adults with cancer and other serious conditions. *Palliative & Supportive Care, 20*(4), pp.462–470.

Wiener, L., McConnell, D.G., Latella, L. and Ludi, E., 2013. Cultural and religious considerations in pediatric palliative care. *Palliative & Supportive Care*, *11*(1), pp. 47–67.
Wiener, L, Zadeh, S, Battles, H, et al., 2012. Allowing adolescents and young adults to plan their end-of-life care. *Pediatrics*, 130, pp. 897–905.
Wiener, L., Zadeh, S., Battles, H., Baird, K., Ballard, E., Osherow, J. and Pao, M., 2012. Allowing adolescents and young adults to plan their end-of-life care. *Pediatrics*, *130*(5), pp. 897–905.
Wright, M., 2020. Dementia, cognitive transformation, and supported decision making. *The American Journal of Bioethics*, *20*(8), pp.88–90.
Yamaguchi, T., Maeda, I., Hatano, Y., Suh, S.Y., Cheng, S.Y., Kim, S.H., Chen, P.J., Morita, T., Tsuneto, S. and Mori, M., 2021. Communication and behavior of palliative care physicians of patients with cancer near end of life in three East Asian countries. *Journal of Pain and Symptom Management*, *61*(2), pp.315–322.
Younge, D., Moreau, P., Ezzat, A. and Gray, A., 1997. Communicating with cancer patients in Saudi Arabia. *Annals of the New York Academy of Sciences*, *809*, pp.309–316.
Zhang, B., Wright, A.A., Huskamp, H.A., Nilsson, M.E., Maciejewski, M.L., Earle, C.C., Block, S.D., Maciejewski, P.K. and Prigerson, H.G., 2009. Health care costs in the last week of life: associations with end-of-life conversations. *Archives of Internal Medicine*, *169*(5), pp.480–488.

5 Meaning making through reflecting on memories, life storying, and legacy leaving

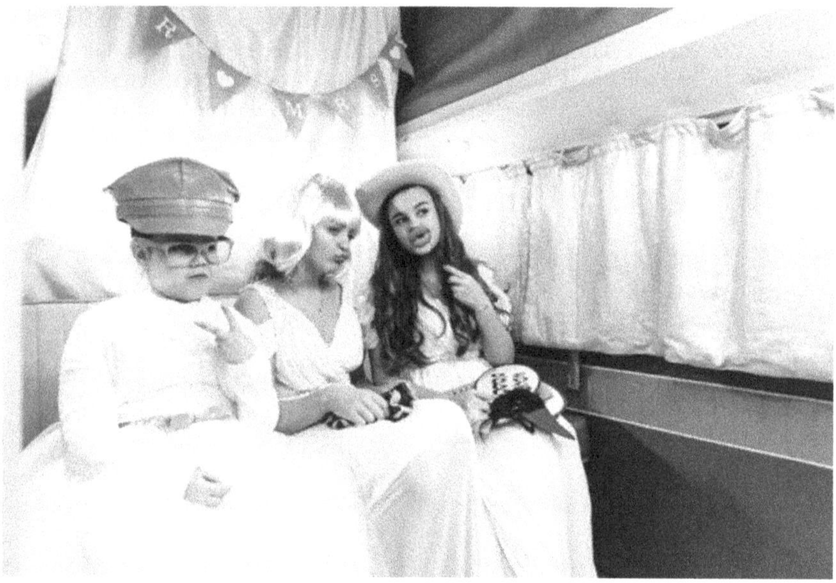

Figure 5.1 A photograph of three young people having a photograph taken in a 'dress up' wedding photobooth.
Photograph taken by Alison Rodriguez.

Introduction

Everyone is different. However, for many individuals approaching the end of their life, there is a natural reflection on what life has meant to them and others, an attempt to make sense of what life has been about. With that reflection can bring some concerns, and a focus on regrets, reasons for emotional unrest and worry. For others, and with support, life can be viewed through a lens of satisfaction. Where individuals can feel some sense of peace and understanding and

DOI: 10.4324/9781003340287-6

an integration of their life experiences, they then do not necessarily fear their death or of talking about it.

Reflecting on the various stages of our lives and the momentous events we have lived through is characteristic of temporal experience and a fundamental aspect of our sense of continuity. The person's life and human experience can be viewed as a whole narrative with a beginning, middle and an end. The story can be read as an edited display of meanings and beliefs (Heidegger, 1962; Ricoeur, 1984). Most of the events that we might place on our 'timeline' are routine. Some, however, mark major changes: marriage, the birth of a child, the death of a parent, retirement. After such events, things are not what they were before. Scannel (2000, p56) when she learned that she might have cancer wrote, *'I felt my life organising into a sharply divided 'before' and 'after', with cancer cleaving the middle'*. The experience of before and after presumes the temporal continuity of our lives, but such news, may not merely indicate a change in life but can also provide a signpost for its closure, for example when an individual is offered end of life care. Such transitions can also signal the end of one's self-identity and the beginning of another.

Putting together a life history or a compilation of certain memories produces a legacy that highlights the personality, accomplishments and often thoughts and desires of its creator. It is also contended that the leaving of something behind relates to image maintenance and an attempt at holding control over how we will be remembered. This is especially poignant when we may be living through a period of life which allows us little or no control. As Bauman (1992) adds, as humans we have an innate desire to be more than the self and our inability to understand nothingness makes us want to strive for post death image management.

The paradoxical nature of our human existence is evident when working within and being in receipt of palliative care, supporting life and death.

Biographical disruption

Biographical disruption is a term that was conceptualised to understand the experience of rheumatoid arthritis. Bury's (1982) original analysis, identified that his participants experienced three main changes in their selves, firstly in their 'taken for granted assumptions and behaviours' (Bury, 1982). Secondly, they were forced to engage in thinking about their futures and how their plans and related identities may change. And thirdly, they had to mobilise resources to cope. Since there have been many authors apply the concept of biographical disruption to their works to enable an understanding of the impact of different diagnoses and the lived experience of different illnesses. Thus, highlighting the strength and utility of the concept.

However, there have also been studies to critique this concept. Williams (2000) suggests for example, that the concept is too simplistic and does not consider the influence of other biographical characteristics on the impact and experience of illness, for example, age and class. Individuals who are diagnosed with a serious illness in older age may not experience the large impacts on identity and the rethinking about the self and the future that young people do, because their expectations of life are already very different and are expectant of deteriorations in health (Adamson and Donovan, 2005). With a similar sentiment, a young person with a serious illness from early childhood may not experience biographical disruption until much later in their disease trajectories because their biographies and self-concepts are already shaped to some extent by their condition (Lowton et al., 2017; Monaghan and Gabe, 2016). This is particularly relevant to young people born with life limiting conditions where there has been no former period of a differently perceived wellness.

Some authors have also highlighted that where people are diagnosed with a serious illness in adolescence then there can be two outcomes.

1. The adolescent plays little attention to the illness and its implications because their focus is on their adolescent development and the developmental tasks relative to adolescent identity formation. In which instances, the impact could be seen more as a biographical contingency (Monaghan and Gabe, 2015). For example, where young people accept that serious illness is now just one component of their identities and their future lives.
2. Being told one has a serious illness at this time of life could be interpreted as a massive blow to the young person's self-identity and future goals and so then the biographical disruption is major. Because identity is fragile in these years, anyway, having to then reconcile key developmental and life goals and be more dependent and less autonomous than peers could impact them psychologically. To these ends, the original concept does not consider the possible magnitude of disruption either (McDonagh et al., 2016).

Class is another mitigating factor. For some individuals they are repeatedly exposed to situations that cause them biographical disruption, not just illness. For those who suffer multiple uncertainties in their lives for example financial instability, difficulty to find and maintain employment, relationship breakdowns, then their lives are a series of disruptions rather than lives marked by one distinct issue (Williams, 2000). A qualitative study exploring the lived experiences of women with HIV identified how some talked about a biographical disruption due to their HIV status and wellness, however others cited life issues such as drug dependence, child separation and domestic violence as more impactful than their illness on their lives. Therefore, it is possible that if an individual's life experience has been filled with disruptions, they may not feel that serious illness has the big biographical disruption that it can have on others (Ciambrone, 2001).

In addition, two further concepts, related to biographical disruption, have been identified: 'biographical suspension' (Bunzli et al., 2013) and 'biographical oscillation' (Bell et al., 2016). Both these concepts could hold relevance for some individuals living with serious illness.

Biographical suspension considers how individuals can tend to put their life on hold until they feel they can reach a time where they can return to the 'real me'. This could be relative to individuals having periods of poor physical symptom control and their coping mechanisms moving their mental focus away from disease progression. This can limit their adaptation to their current or developing health status because their belief is that their current health state is temporary (Bunzli et al., 2013). In addition, Sanders (2015) suggests the non linear nature of some serious illnesses requires a process of adaptation and re-adaptation, rather than a reactive adaptation to an event that we interpret as highly stressful. Indeed, for many individuals with serious illness, it is a process of 'normalisation' that they engage with, combining aspects of their new situation into pre-existing narratives of their lives and selves. To some extent this could be an alternative view of the impact of serious illness in people's lives. Sanderson et al. (2011) identify that the concept of biographical disruption negates normalisation a common shared feature of illness experience.

It may also be possible that through the highs and lows of living with serious illness, individuals experience a 'biographical oscillation', in that they move from periods of disruption to normalisation and vice versa, at different points in their disease trajectories (Bell et al., 2016). Many congenital life limiting conditions involve acute episodes which disturb an otherwise normal lifestyle, shifting the individual's focus to the aspects of themselves which are implicated with/by illness. What Bury did identify was that non-communicable diseases do not 'break-out', they 'creep up'. Acute episodes in the context of life limiting illness can bring about biographical change, bringing the individuals' attention more focused on the nature and limits of their condition, but this may still not be perceived as a biographical disruption. When a life limiting condition has flares of ill health, or poor symptom management, then these episodes are not so much disruption but confirmation, a reminder that the individual's authentic biography is one of being an individual with a serious illness. Sometimes acute events or disease exacerbations can also bring about a sense of belonging – to disease communities, validating identity and removing any scepticism. Alternatively, where conditions are life threatening and begin following years of good health, then the condition does reconfigure life for them.

Meaning making in serious illness

The search for meaning in serious illness is a complex and continuous process. Studies have often situated their focus on adjustment or adaptation to conditions. However, when the condition is life threatening or life limiting, the adjustment is not just to a different state of health but may involve a reframing of life goals and longer lifetime plans (Pinquart et al., 2009). The process of change in outlook can be spiritual, with deterioration can come existential concern and then more weight is placed on the need to make sense and meaning out of the illness and what is happening. Researchers appreciate the subjective nature of meaning making in this context and through appreciation of the individuals lived experiences and perceptions, health and social care professionals can then better provide person centred rather than disease focused care (Irwin and Richardson, 2006).

Meaning making in reaction to a knowledge of the relative immediacy of dying is not well understood, however the psychological exercise appears to impact positively on several psychosocial outcomes, such as quality of life factors. As such there is argument that meaning making is a measurable concept (Steger et al., 2006). From a theoretical perspective, Frankl (1947/2021) suggested that it is our human nature to find meaning and the human pursuit of life involves purposeful and goal focused action. From a social psychological position, Bandura (1986) developed Frankl's thinking and argued that in fact all human behaviour is driven by meaning and goals, especially in times of stress. Frankl's work on meaning making has since been conceptualised as global meaning, which gives humans direction in their lives (Lazarus and Folkman, 1984). Global meaning includes the connections we have to things and others that give human meaning, which relate to belief systems, future expectations, and subjective emotionality.

Behaviours, thoughts or emotions that are attached to meanings influence our perceptions of our life situations. New meanings however can evolve through the desire for a sense of calm and to lessen feelings of anxiety. Sherman et al. (2010) conducted research with participants recently diagnosed with life threatening illness. They found an association between global meaning and distress. When global meaning increased, distress decreased and perceptions of quality of life also increased. In addition, Skeath et al. (2013) undertook a qualitative exploration of individual's aggressive life limiting conditions and their perceptions of meaning making and healing. Where participants reported subjective healing, psychosocial or spiritual suffering was reduced.

Leaving a legacy

A body of research is growing that has explored how legacy making can assist meaning making in palliative and end of life care. Various stipulations exist regarding what a legacy or leaving a legacy means (Boles and Jones, 2021). The use of the word legacy in terms of will making is commonplace and therefore legacy in this sense relates to the passing on of financial or material possessions to others in the event of our deaths. Legacy can take different forms but there is a consensus that it involves the passing on of something or of leaving something behind for others (Hunter, 2008). It can also be that legacies are passed on at various times of life and not just when one is dying or has died (Allen, 2008). The passing on of traditions is a legacy, for example, families using the same baptism gown for each young child in the family is a shared legacy. Indeed, legacy or the creation of a legacy could be both an individual and shared enterprise.

Creating and transmitting a legacy is also one way an individual can conclude their life story and manage their identities. Legacies expressed in a life story format can also be shared with future generations. In this way, a legacy can detail the individual's life.

Our human nature influences how we categorise the events of our lives into past, present and future, beginning, middle or end. By doing so we can appreciate our worldly experiences, our contributions to life and other's world views (Bruner, 2002).

Our life experiences are situated in time and space and in relationships and we draw on narratives to be able to connect to our different worldviews (Heidegger, 1962; Ricoeur, 1984). When we share our experiences, we do so recounting the temporal and spatial qualities that stories allow. Our stories are much more than a sequence of happenings, they are enriched with expressions of temporality, spatiality and relationality.

McAdams' (1996) life story model of identity suggests that individuals narrate their self through their experiences. This gives their lives meaning and purpose. He argues that identity is a story of the self, and the story harnesses the complexities of our human interactions and feelings. The life story is therefore also an expression of our values, and the narrative says as much about the teller and their identity as it does the events of their lives. Our life stories are forever edited with each telling and each cultural context. We position ourselves as unique and the story is told with a moral framework and items are denied inclusion if they overshadow the key messages we want to promote. In creating a coherent life story, we begin to consider its conclusion, how we want to live to our death, and the ways we would like to be remembered.

Psychological development considerations

McAdams (1996) work promotes the innate value of the life story which is congruent with Erikson's (1968) adult life stages of generativity and ego integrity. The generativity versus stagnation stage of this theory details the human need to leave something of our lives to society and for future generations. Ego integrity versus despair is the labelled process of making sense of one's life when the end of one's life is in closer view. Life stages necessitate identity work. Towards the end of our lives our life stories are made prominent in our minds for reflection and an opportunity of time is provided to reconceptualise some of our life chapters (Coleman, 1999).

Erikson's idea of 'generativity' has been described as a biological phenomenon (reproduction), a philosophical or religious perspective (transcendence and immortality), a developmental task (normal growth), and a societal demand (source of productivity) (McAdams, 1996; McAdams et al., 1993). McAdams' subsequent theory of generativity identifies that the need for generativity is something creative to our cultural and social connectedness and inner desires. Our motivation for generativity is to have had purpose in life but also purpose beyond death. Through generativity we can keep hold of the notable events in our lives, the important aspects of ourselves, and share them. The ultimate feature of McAdams' generativity is the story telling or our narrative. Generativity is a big element of our life story. Our identities evolve through that life story (McAdams, 1996). Generativity itself is a script in the overall story, reflecting particularly how we see ourselves and how we want others to view us.

John Kotre (1984) mused a lot over the concept of generativity. For Kotre, generativity is about maintenance of the self and creating a self that will transcend death. He also delineated types of generativities and suggested that it is cultural generativity that holds most prominence for the self. This type emerges when the person can appreciate an understanding, a belongingness and responsibility to pass on items of wisdom or value. To engage with this process, the individual needs to appreciate that they are a part of a larger system of meaning. We strive to understand this meaning when we are trying to understand the end of our lives.

Although generativity is identified as something that is poignant to middle age, earlier psychosocial development can have episodes of generative thinking. For example, Lawford et al. (2020) in a longitudinal study of community involvement found generative thinking in young people aged 14 to 16 years. Those with an interest in legacy also displayed prosocial behaviours and secure attachment styles. With this shared desire for generativity across age groups it is possible that meaning making and legacy leaving is relative for all individuals with serious illness and their families and that tailored interventions have a place to play in their psycho-social and spiritual support and wellbeing.

Generativity, meaning making and legacy: psychotherapeutic interventions

Despite the holistic philosophy of palliative care there is a dearth of research studies that explore the need, development, and efficacy of psychotherapeutic interventions for individuals of different ages with different conditions and their families (Gibson and Breitbart, 2004). Health and social care professionals, even those working in palliative care can also sometimes not acknowledge the benefit psychotherapeutic intervention can have for individuals with serious illness and advancing disease (Rodin and Gillies, 2009).

The small developing literature base is very much dictated by approaches that are spiritual in their content. For example, they range from yoga-based practices to Buddhist techniques of meditation to interventions that reflect on self-transcendence and Viktor Frankl's logotherapy that is spiritually meaning making based.

Therapeutic life review

One psychotherapeutic intervention is called therapeutic life review and has been developed from an intervention that was originally designed for the prevention and management of depression in older adults (Mastel-Smith et al., 2006). This therapeutic intervention is based on Erikson's stages of psychosocial development; the final two stages of generativity versus stagnation and ego integrity versus despair. There are several stages to the intervention. In adapting the intervention for individuals in receipt of palliative care it was realised that the latter stages of the intervention may hold most worth. It is in these stages that the life of the individual is looked over and the individual comes to accept, sometimes with guidance that their life has had meaning and value. According to Erikson if we do not achieve this understanding of our lives then we can become focused on the events of life that can induce guilt and emotional torment (Erikson, 1968).

The act of reflection helps us to put our life events into perspective and to depict what events have impacted on the wellbeing of ourselves and others. By doing this we can begin to engender a sense of peace over the life we have lived and be open to live through our concluding chapter (Haber, 2006). Therapeutic life review has been drawn upon using different techniques, for example in counselling sessions, through creating written biographies and engaging in focused life review interviews (Lloyd-Williams et al., 2013).

Several studies, conducted in the USA, Canada and Asia have explored the effectiveness of this intervention on different measurable wellbeing outcomes and has shown benefits for individuals, especially those with advanced cancer conditions (Breitbart et al., 2012).

The outlook intervention

The outlook intervention is a life review-oriented intervention (Steinhauser et al., 2008). The main purpose of it is to help the individual with serious illness to explore their existential/spiritual needs by looking back on their lives and considering which parts of their lives or what events they would like to relive or change in some way. This helps individuals to see what fun they have had in life and to see that even in tough times there may have been some benefit. This process can also help them to set future goals, redoing things they feel they need to redo and experiencing things that might help them reflect with a more positive lens and support important future decision making. This intervention has a distinct structure that requires the facilitator or therapist to conduct three 60-minute sessions with the individual. There are fixed questions and prompt cards, and the sessions are digitally recorded. At the close of each session there is also time set aside for the individual to sit in quiet contemplation to reflect further on the content of that session.

Unlike some other meaning making interventions, a legacy product is not created. However, because the sessions are digitally recorded these can be transcribed and hard copies given to individuals if desired.

The outlook intervention questions include:

- Session 1: The Life Story Session – Tell me about your life? What are your cherished times? Of what are you most proud? If someone were to make a movie of your life, what would be important to include?

- Session 2: The Forgiveness Session – If you were to do things again, what might you do differently? Are there things or times you regret? Is there anyone to whom you would like to offer forgiveness? Is there anyone from whom you would like to ask forgiveness? Are you at peace?
- Session 3: The Heritage & Legacy Session – What are your most valuable lessons learned? What would you like to share with future generations? If you could choose one thing to pass on as your legacy what would that be? What things would you like to accomplish? (Steinhauser et al., 2008)

The first outlook session gets individuals to think about their lives lived to date and to recall the events of their past which they recount as holding the most importance to them. This is also the major gist of the original life review intervention (Haber, 2006). The prompt cards are used with the individual to help them recall their stories. For example, there are cards that suggest thinking about family, their childhood, certain people and places. This session can allude to the positive and the negative memories. Where there was past tensions or deflations the therapist collaborates with the individual to hold those events for session two. In session two the individual is guided to reconsider those more negative events and to think about if there are any ways now that those memories could be reconceptualised, or the events be revisited to put issues to rest. In wider studies, forgiveness has been identified as contributory to the healing process (Waltman et al., 2009) and it is in this session that individuals are invited to forgive others and themselves for errors on their life path. In the final session the individual is invited to consider messages they would like to generate for their significant others following their death. Again, the prompt cards can be used to think about how this could be achieved. Individuals can engage for example in scrap booking or letter writing at this juncture. It is in this session that the individual is also asked to think about their own future life goals. People with serious illness still have lives to live and may have considered many opportunities they want to fulfil, having a support network to verbalise these wishes can help them to start thinking about how they can go about operationalising them (Chochinov, 2004, Chochinov et al., 2005). Goal setting can also provide hope and thus lessen feelings of depression and death related anxiety (Breitbart et al., 2000).

Memory banking

In keeping with the understanding that life storying can be of psychotherapeutic benefit, especially for those at the end of their lives, a further intervention has been developed called Memory Banking (MB). In retracing and narrating the life story, individuals convey memories of people, places and events that each can engender accompanied sensation, emotion, behaviour, decisions and worldviews (van Manen, 1990). The MB intervention was originally developed to combine five activities that are validated reducing age related distress and burden. These activities include:

1. Life story development
2. Communication
3. Social support
4. Brain exercise and
5. Legacy building.

Studies evidence that when individuals engage in narrative life history interviews, they find much pleasure in doing so and there are noted benefits to improvements in mental health status (Hilgeman et al., 2014). The intervention encourages a lot of talking and being listened to and being involved in questioning, offered by an active listener. Communication therefore is supportive in this context and in studies has shown that where individuals are feeling lonely and have little opportunity to socialise, that time for day-to-day dialogue, and active communication can improve health outcomes (Chung, 2009). The support felt can also lessen the person's sense of burden and distress (Chiang, et al., 2010). This 'together talking' can feel socially supportive and an increased sense of social support (Spitznagel et al., 2006). The social nature of the intervention, involving a group sharing of reminiscence can also promote interpersonal and social connections with others (Perese et al., 2008).

The intervention can be particularly useful for those struggling with memory loss because both the structure of the brain and its functioning can benefit from trying to remember notable events and in sequencing memories. This can become a more fluent activity with repeated practice (Swaab et al., 2002). In a bid to fully explore episodic memory (that contains memories linked to subjective experiences as related to time, events, and places) (Papalia et al., 2007) the intervention takes the individual through a string of activities that are complimented by visual imagery, spoken and written words and a chunking of life information. At the close of the intervention, legacies are situated within the stories told (Hunter and Rowles, 2005).

The process of the legacy is driven by the life story. Both the legacy and the life story combined give meaning to experiences, help people to understand themselves and others better. The MB intervention helps individuals to think about and construe their legacies and with clarity. It may be the first time that they can look back on their lives and see that it has had meaning and purpose and that their value continues in their current lives and future plans (Hunter and Rowles, 2005).

These types of interventions are also beneficial for palliative care practice and professional understanding of the individuals and families in their care. The individual's situation can be viewed in the context of their lives. It is with this information that the individual can be viewed as so much more than their presenting condition or age.

Logotherapy

Logotherapy emanates from the seminal work of Victor Frankl (1947/2021). The essence of the therapy is conceptualised around how individuals always want control over themselves, and their own behaviours and it does not matter what conditions are placed upon them, this need for control prevails.

Logotherapy aims to decrease individuals' suffering and to allow individuals to have the opportunity to live their lives to their fullest. This is achieved by supporting individuals to do activities that make them think about their meaning and purpose in life. The wider work of Frank has one major theme: *'The longing to find meaning within the content of our lives and within our existence is not just mere coincidence but, rather, is a primary motivating force within humans'* (Frankl, 1947/2021). The understanding is that life always has meaning, right up until the point we die.

Logotherapy has developed on from existential analysis, otherwise termed existential therapy (Frankl, 1947/2021). Logotherapy just concentrates on meaning where therapists encourage individuals to explore meaning 'through "creative values," "experiential values," and "attitudinal values"' (Ameli and Dattilio, 2013).

Several therapy driven techniques are used to achieve this meaning:

1. Paradoxical intention: like exposure therapy, the individual is encouraged to keep reflecting on something that has worried them or something they have feared, and the situation is reconceptualised with humour.
2. Dereflection: based on 'self-transcendence', the individual is encouraged to move attention from negative aspects of life to what is positive in their life, e.g., those who love and care for them.
3. Attitude modification: rather than focusing on thoughts this technique is focused on attitude change. For example, if the individual is suffering with anticipatory grief, they may be encouraged to think more positive about bereavement.

Logotherapy's focus is to adopt new ways of thinking and acting to make individuals' worlds more meaningful.

Meaning centred group psychotherapy

Meaning centered group psychotherapy (MCP) also aims to assist individuals (people with cancer) manage their meaning making and to find peace and purpose in life (Breitbart et al., 2010). The intervention involves both a therapeutic attitude involving instruction and discussion but also experiential exercises. Eight group sessions are actioned under the following specific meaning-centred themes:

Session 1. Summary of concepts and sources of meaning
Session 2. Cancer and meaning

Sessions 3 and 4. Meaning derived from the historical context of life
Session 5. Meaning derived from attitudinal values
Session 6. Meaning derived from creative values and responsibility
Session 7. Meaning derived through experiential values
Session 8. Termination and feedback.

Lichtenthal et al. (2020) further explore the theoretical framework underlying MCP inspired by the work of Frankl (1947/2021) and Irvin Yalom (1980/2020). They provide a case vignette as detailed in Box 5.1 to show how the approach can work in practice.

Box 5.1 Case Vignette (Lichtenthal et al., 2020, p24)

'Dr X was a 40-year-old, married physician with one child who began MCP shortly after he received a diagnosis of advanced pancreatic cancer. Though sceptical of how "meaning" could help him, Dr X was hoping for relief from the overwhelming distress he was experiencing about his diagnosis. He was particularly upset by changes in his ability to work as a physician and fulfil responsibilities to his wife, children, and aging parents.

During Session 2, Identity Before and After Cancer, it became clear that being suddenly thrust into the patient role threatened Dr X's sense of identity as someone who provides care for others and strives for perfection. While Dr X acknowledged gaining a greater understanding of the existential nature of his distress through discussion, he expressed frustration that there was no way to "fix" this suffering.

In Session 3, Historical Sources of Meaning, the concept of legacy proved to be the key to shifting the meaning Dr X made of his current struggles. He realised the distress around perceived changes to his identity were connected to the legacy he was given, as he had been encouraged by his family to be perfect and "fix things." He realized he could choose to respond differently to the legacy he was given, leading to changes in how he parented and allowing things to be imperfect and "messy" more often.

As sessions progressed, ways that Dr X creatively responded to the physical challenges he faced were identified, reinforcing the concepts of choice and courage in how he faced his predicament. This included the choice to engage in MCP despite his scepticism and to accept help from others, which became a meaningful lesson he wanted to model for his child. In his final session, Dr X expressed feeling more connected to the people who mattered most to him, recognizing new ways he could continue to share his legacy of responsibility and caregiving with those whose lives he touched personally and professionally'.

The intervention uses social support to encourage healing and to help individuals with their peers, confront their existential challenges presented by a life-threatening illness. So far, the therapeutic intervention has been developed for those with cancer conditions and has been trialled with good outcomes observed on a range of quality-of-life dimensions (Breitbart, 2010; Breitbart et al., 2015).

Dignity Therapy

Dignity Therapy (DT) for individuals with serious illness was developed by Harvey Max Chochinov and colleagues, following a depth of qualitative work with older adults with cancer, which had influenced the dignity conserving model of care (DCMC). This dignity conserving model of care is a guide for meeting the dignity needs of individuals living with serious illness. Both this model and subsequently, DT, although it was first designed for the use for individuals with cancer, has been found to be relevant to individuals with a range of serious illnesses (Chochinov et al., 2005; Chochinov, 2012).

DT aims to address individuals' psychosocial and existential distress via a one-to-one focused interview. It is a brief and individualised psychotherapeutic intervention that has been designed to engender a sense of meaning and purpose for the person who is facing the end of their life (Chochinov, et al., 2005).

During DT, a discussion is held around nine key questions (see Box 5.2) between the individual and a DT trained professional. The questions encourage a life reflection, they engage the individual in the recalling of memories and encourage them to think about and verbalise their hopes and wishes for others. Collectively this is a process that is a pursuit to meaning make about their life and purpose and for them to develop a legacy for others. The session will usually last for around one hour and is recorded for later transcription. Following transcription, the therapist edits the document into a cohesive narrative that is then checked by the individual and with the assistance of the therapist, final edits are made. This document is the individual's generativity document, their written legacy. Individuals then choose to bequeath the document to a person or persons of their choosing, before or after their death.

Over time, and as more professionals have been trained in the approach there has been some adjustments made to how the legacy document is presented. For example, in collaborating with people with limited cognitive capacity, the legacy documents have evolved into picture books, including cherished photos alongside briefer commentaries (Montross et al., 2011). The sharing of these documents has also provided families with the opportunities for meaningful conversations, assisting bereavement processes (McClement, et al., 2007).

DT is being used globally with adults and the outcome data of trials has so far suggested there can be benefit to measures of adult wellbeing and overall quality of life (Chochinov et al., 2005; Chochinov, 2012).

Box 5.2 The Dignity Therapy Question Protocol (Chochinov, 2012)

Dignity Therapy Question Protocol

1. Tell me a little about your life history, particularly the parts that you either remember most or think are the most important? When did you feel most alive?
2. Are there specific things that you would want your family to know about you, and are there particular things you would want them to remember?
3. What are the most important roles you have played in life (family roles, vocational roles, community service roles, etc.)? Why were they so important to you and what do you think you accomplished in those roles?
4. What are your most important accomplishments, and what do you feel most proud of?
5. Are there particular things that you feel still need to be said to your loved ones, or things that you would want to take the time to say once again?
6. What are your hopes and dreams for your loved ones?
7. What have you learned about life that you would want to pass along to others? What advice or words of guidance would you wish to pass along to your [son, daughter, husband, wife, parents, other(s)]?
8. Are there words or perhaps even instructions you would like to offer your family, to help prepare them for the future?
9. In creating this permanent record, are there other things that you would like included?

Dignity Therapy for young people

A rapid structured evidence review was undertaken to explore the use of DT and other meaning making interventions with young people in palliative care (Rodriguez et al., 2018). It was identified that current research trials of DT have been void of including individuals below the age of 25 years, regardless of condition group. However, four studies highlighted some participation in adult trials of the original DT and one study included a videography adapted version of DT for adolescents with cancer (Akard et al., 2015). These works suggested that DT may prove beneficial for young people with life limiting conditions.

Since this review, several studies have been undertaken to undertake DT with young people. Juliao et al. (2020a,b) have adapted the questions of the original DT protocol via a professional consensus method for adolescents with cancer and are embarking on feasibility studies to evaluate the acceptability of the approach with young people in Portugal. A digital story board technique, again for adolescents with cancer and based upon DT, has also been recently trialled with success by Akard et al. (2020) in Tennessee, USA. In addition, Schuelke and Rubenstein (2020), Texas USA, have developed a hospital based flexible approach to using original DT with children and young people, undertaken by proxy with families where needed (for those preverbal or nonverbal). They report some hesitance amongst families and health professionals in selecting young people to participate in the approach but illustrate beneficial outcomes, for example:

> *'Miracle Akbar was a 16-year-old girl who was diagnosed with metastatic alveolar rhabdomyosarcoma. Before her death, Miracle began creating legacy items for her mother and six siblings, which made her an excellent candidate for Dignity Therapy. Miracle's disease affected her ability to speak, which made recording her interview difficult. The recording was successfully transcribed from a whisper. Her story contained significant hardship and tragedy, and the authors had concerns it may not be therapeutic for her to hear it retold. When Miracle's story was read back to her, she replied back with a firm, "It's perfect." Miracle wished for a party before she died. At that party, she read her completed Dignity Therapy document to everyone who attended and subsequently reported with a wry smile, "Everyone cried. It was great."'*
>
> *'Shahd Shahroor is a 20-year-old girl with cystic fibrosis. When Shahd was 17, she had rapidly progressive respiratory failure. She acknowledged that her life may end soon and wanted to leave a strong legacy behind her. She loved telling stories, so Dignity Therapy was very much in line with her goals and personality. Her parents spoke Arabic, and her wish was for her story to be sent back to Palestine after she died. With that in mind, the document was translated to Arabic to achieve Shahd's wish. Remarkably, Shahd was able to receive a lung transplant. She is currently living at home with her family, enjoying her newfound time. She feels "excited" hearing where her document has been shared for educational purposes'.*

These studies alongside consultation activities, including twitter chats with young people, families and professionals, closed Facebook groups with young people with serious illness and professional workshops have established support for the further amendment and development of DT for young people with serious illness (Watts et al., 2019, 2020a, 2020b). The consultation activities suggested that DT in its current format is not so attractive to younger people with serious illness, the questions need reframing to be more reflective of young people's lives and for those who have lived with serious illness from early childhood especially. In addition, there was suggestion that a more motivational and inclusive DT based intervention for young people with serious illness would be delivered in a digital format. An application that could draw on young people's creativity and include the arts, for example, with facilities to upload artwork and music would be welcomed. As a result, studies are currently underway, to co-create with young people with serious illness, their families and health and social care professionals, a DT based digital intervention that will be called DIGNISPACE (Rodriguez et al., forthcoming). In the first instance, this application will be developed for young people with life limiting conditions aged 18 to 24 years. The expectation, however, is that over time the intervention will be further developed for a wider age range of young people with serious illness and their families.

Societal meaning making and the death café movement

Meaning making, generativity and legacy making packaged within psychotherapeutic interventions encourage us to think about death and dying, so we can try and make our last life chapter more purposeful. It is not until we get to this stage however, that we usually open our hearts and minds to this stage of our lives. The death café movement has a therapeutic basis, in drawing on shared focused conversation and has the aim to engage communities in a shared openness about death and dying, to provide a means for social and informational support around death (please also see Chapter 7 the good death for reference to the death positivity movement and other community-based initiatives promoting an openness around talk about death and dying).

Death Cafes are recreational community events usually devoted to raising awareness about death, dying and grief (Miles and Corr, 2017). Groups of 20–30 people gather around with coffee/tea and biscuits/cake for 2 hours of so and discuss matters to do with facing their own death (and what to do if and when that happens); bereavement and grief (what to do for others; what to expect from your own experiences of losses); the status of death and dying in communities, neighbourhoods, or workplaces today, and so on. The cafes are opportunities to learn from each other's experiences, to explore a commonly 'taboo' topic and to learn about one's own needs before a crisis makes them obvious.

The history of death café

On 23 March 2004, Bernard Crettaz (2010) the Swiss sociologist and anthropologist held his first Café Mortel in Switzerland. Following on from this initial café he hosted a further forty cafes before his retirement. He also published *Café mortels: Sortir mort du silence*, a book about his experience of death café.

A British web designer, Jon Underwood, decided that there was continued work to be done in this arena and picked up the torch of what we now know as the death café movement. In September 2011, Underwood hosted his first death cafe with Sue Barsky Reid, a psychotherapist. On his death cafe website, he reported that the café was attended by six people with diverse backgrounds including a nun and a management consultant. Later in January 2012, Underwood co-hosted a Death Cafe gathering in conjunction with Southbank Death: Festival for the Living, more affectionately known as Death Fest. The cafe was well received and since we have seen death cafes occurring throughout the UK and increasingly in the USA.

The first death café in the USA was July 2012, attendees were asked to write a small note of their reason of attendance (Miles and Corr, 2017 (see Box 5.3 to 5.8 for noted reasons of attendance).

Box 5.3 Example 1 reason to attend death café

Example 1: Processing loss related to own mortality

My brother-in-law died this past April and my husband, and I have been thinking a lot about his life and how it had not been a fulfilling one for him. How his brother did not actually do the things he said he wanted to do. Which, in turn, has made us think a lot about our own lives and plans. We have both worked in hospice and would very much like to attend the next meeting.

Box 5.4 Example 2 reason to attend death café

Example 2: Processing loss as a metaphysical experience

I read the article in the paper and found the thought of this gathering intriguing. I have only lost a few people in my life so far and of those losses I have had interesting experiences with two of them that have made me feel confident that there is something else for us after we pass away. I would be interested to hear what other people have to say about their experiences and acceptance of death. While I can at least think about my loved ones that have since now passed without crying, their loss still saddens me, and I would like to see if others may have found better and or different ways to cope. I did not find traditional grief counselling very helpful and thought this opportunity might help me cope in some way. I have a tendency to observe more than share in a group setting, but if the group tends to be animated, I would probably share what I consider unusual experiences.

Box 5.5 Example 3 reason to attend death café

Example 3: Examining the mortality of loved ones

Hi there! I'm interested in attending this event because I'm an only child, technically speaking (I don't speak with my biological father or his other children). My mom and step-dad are all I have, and they are both getting older and live on the East Coast. My step-dad in particular has a family history of heart attacks and strokes, and just last year there was a major scare when a tree came down just a few feet from their home during a hurricane. I realized then that I wouldn't know how to handle the inevitable, and both my parents are unwilling to discuss it. So, perhaps something like this will get me comfortable with it and, in turn, help them get comfortable with it!

Box 5.6 Example 4 reason to attend death café

Example 4: Academic/Philosophical

I'm very intrigued and would be very enthusiastic about attending the first Death Cafe here in Columbus. My interest in death and attending is largely academic, but also philosophical. The oft-repeated phrase about nothing staying the same except for death and taxes is really quite an apt description. I find it bizarre for such a universal experience to not be shared more openly. I also would like to challenge my own preconceptions of death, and hopefully expand the meaning and scope of my life by having a better understanding of death and dying. My schedule is clear for that evening, and I hope my presence would make the event more enriched. I hope to hear more as the event draws near.

Box 5.7 Example 5 reason to attend death café

Example 5: Desire to Help Others

I am 50 years old and have been widowed twice. Both of my husbands passed away via suicide. The first time in 1983 when I was 20 and the second time in 2007 when I was 45. Grieving and learning to live again is something that I know well. If I can, I would like to come to listen and offer my perspective. I look forward to hearing from you!

Box 5.8 Example 6 reason to attend death café

Example 6: Professional

I'm a hospice nurse. I've been at it for 25 years. I would love to come and visit with people. I'm obviously a strong advocate for early intervention'.

These examples identify the breadth of interest in the death café movement and how commonly interest does arise from those already bereaved, seeking comfort and answers. However, there is always a disclaimer that death café is not 'a bereavement support group'. Still much learning can arise from the relaxed discussion that happenings in the death café setting.

The death café gives value to human sharing and context for death related discussion. Kastenbaum (2000) in 'The Psychology of Death' suggested that we have a death system in every society and that each system has a network that has systems which function to mediate death with members. For example, in the western death system we have police officers, emergency care professions, palliative care professionals, medical examiners and coroners, funeral homes and cemeteries, funerals, memorials, public memorials, symbolised death using hearses, certain discourse etc. Palliative care plays its part in this death system and with time we welcome newcomers. The death café has joined this framework of support highlighting our death social systems are as dynamic as our heath care systems.

Digital meaning making and grief legacy

Since the industrial revolution, the internet has commanded the biggest social changes of our age, influencing how we work and how we share information. Recent Ofcom statistics highlight that in the UK individuals spend on average 22.9 hours a week online, with those aged 16–24 spending 35.2 hours a week online. This online presence involves social media usage interacting with platforms such as Facebook, Instagram, TikTok, and Twitter, sharing opinion, stories, photographs and videos. This communication method enables our voices to be heard across boundaries of distance and age. Indeed, we are becoming digital beings with our digital online presences becoming ingrained in our day to day lives and legacies. Not only do we live a lot of our lives online when we die, we leave our digital lives online. What we leave behind on these digital platforms is conceptualised as our digital legacies (Gulotta et al., 2013).

Social media profiles of the dead continue to exist alongside profiles of the living. The bereaved can continue to manage these accounts and continue to converse with the others their loved ones were connected to in life. For some people, this ongoing mediated conversation with the dead provides comfort and meaning.

As a reaction to this, many online providers have begun to offer post-death digital asset management (Sofka, 2020). It is important that professionals working in palliative care acknowledge the digital lives of individuals and families. Even more so when having advanced planning discussions. For some individuals, just having their password for their mobile device noted down before losing the ability to do so can be of great emotional benefit to the family that is later bereaved. James Norris has established the Digital Legacy Association. This is now the governing organisation responsible for improving the quality of end-of-life care in all areas relating to the protection of digital assets and digital legacy. There is now also the scope for individuals to document their social media wishes in a social media will.

Those born after 2000 have always lived digitally connected lives. A lifetime of living in the digital world necessitates digital end of life planning and meaning making to consider the value of digital assets.

Chapter summary

When an individual is told they have a serious illness or in times of living with a life limiting condition from birth or early years, there can be an array of impacts on the individuals thinking. An acute feeling of stress over how they will cope with their condition. There can be a coming to terms with a changed outlook, and a musing over how they can manage future life goals and wishes. For years within the literature there has been reference made to the concept of biographical disruption that embraces the individuals' reactions and life changes that emanate as the result of a serious illness diagnosis or life shortening prognosis or advancing disease. Serious illness can disrupt lives and outlooks, but the experience can be more nuanced, for some there can be times of putting life on hold to get through episodes of care, treatment difficulties or low mood. This has been conceptualised as biographical suspension. For others or at other times, there can be a biographical oscillation, in they can experience phases of illness that can be highly stressful and emotionally disruptive and then return to phase of normalisation where their identities and self-concepts are integrative of their condition. The way we experience illness and related disruptions can also be impacted by demographic factors such as age and class (of course issues of culture and gender are also relevant but not discussed in any depth within this chapter).

Our developmental trajectories may also influence our desire for reflection, memory making, life storying, meaning making and legacy. In living with serious and advancing illness there becomes a point where the individual wants to engage in life review and consider what words of wisdom or messages they can share about their lives and the wishes they have for others before they die. They also want reassurance that they have had meaning and purpose in their lives.

An array of psychosocial interventions are available to support individuals and families for generativity and meaning making. These have been successfully adapted for condition types and age groups. However, the intervention literature highlights less formalised or tailored interventions for children and young people within palliative needs. There is also a dearth of literature that addresses interventions for young people with neurodegenerative conditions and their families.

In reflecting back to the public health palliative care movement in Chapter 1 it is possible to see the benefits here of a more cultural openness toward death and dying and a more engaged community support network for those with serious illness and advancing disease and their families. Communities can assist openness about death and dying in using strategies such as death café and sharing awareness of social media and digital support and legacy. Communities can also be active in supporting memory making, life reflection and meaning making. This may be as simple as offering support to a family to meet some of the bucket list wishes of their serious ill family member that will enable their legacy.

Key issues

1. As individuals experience serious illness and live through their disease trajectories, they may aim to normalise life with their illness but at times there will be a sense of biographical disruption.
2. With an awareness of living a life shortening prognosis, individuals can benefit from life review and meaning making.

3. Individuals go through developmental stages where generativity is a normative desire, regardless of proximity to death. There are stages of life where individuals have an innate desire to leave something behind for others in a legacy.
4. Life storying can be of emotional benefit for both individuals with serious illness and their families, to explore changes, challenges and assets in their lives.
5. Interventions that have been developed to support memory making, life storying, meaning making and legacy leaving have shown benefits to individuals' quality of life and mood. Families have also reported benefit to later experiences of bereavement.
6. These interventions also engage individuals and health and social care professionals in effective communication processes that can allow for adjunct conversations about both tough and trivial topics. Some may benefit from the social interaction that these interventions bring, lifting them out of feelings of loneliness. In addition, young people can also benefit from having their voice heard and the openness to allow them to talk about what is happening and what their wishes may be.

Box 5.9 Reflective questions

1. In experiencing acute illnesses and for some, long term conditions, there can be a sense of biographical disruption. Does this experience help you to understand the experience of serious illness? Can you appreciate why individuals may engage with the coping mechanisms they do? To both normalise their lives and to continue to find purpose?
2. In hospice care it is commonplace for individuals with serious illness to engage in creativity activities. The outputs of these activities can be kept as meaningful souvenirs for both individuals and their families. Do you think there would be benefit for individuals to have dialogue with others around memories and meaning making? Do you think it is possible for creative pursuits to be used in a more formal legacy project or intervention with children and young people?

References

Adamson, J. and Donovan, J., 2005. 'Normal disruption': South Asian and African/Caribbean relatives caring for an older family member in the UK. *Social Science & Medicine*, *60*(1), pp.37–48.

Akard, T.F., Dietrich, M.S., Friedman, D.L., Hinds, P.S., Given, B., Wray, S. and Gilmer, M.J., 2015. Digital storytelling: An innovative legacy-making intervention for children with cancer. *Pediatric Blood & Cancer*, *62*(4), pp.658–665.

Akard, T.F., Wray, S., Friedman, D.L., Dietrich, M.S., Hendricks-Ferguson, V., Given, B., Gerhardt, C.A., Hinds, P.S. and Gilmer, M.J., 2020. Transforming a face-to-face legacy intervention to a web-based legacy intervention for children with advanced cancer. *Journal of Hospice and Palliative Nursing: JHPN: The Official Journal of the Hospice and Palliative Nurses Association*, *22*(1), p.49.

Allen, R.S., Hilgeman, M.M., Ege, M.A., Shuster Jr, J.L. and Burgio, L.D., 2008. Legacy activities as interventions approaching the end of life. *Journal of Palliative Medicine*, *11*(7), pp.1029–1038.

Ameli, M. and Dattilio, F.M., 2013. Enhancing cognitive behavior therapy with logotherapy: Techniques for clinical practice. *Psychotherapy*, *50*(3), p.387.

Bandura, A., 1986. The explanatory and predictive scope of self-efficacy theory. *Journal of Social and Clinical Psychology*, *4*(3), pp.359–373.

Bauman, Z., 1992. *Mortality, Immortality and Other Life Strategies*. Stanford University Press.

Bell, S.L., Tyrrell, J. and Phoenix, C., 2016. Ménière's disease and biographical disruption: where family transitions collide. *Social Science & Medicine*, *166*, pp.177–185.

Boles, J.C. and Jones, M.T., 2021. Legacy perceptions and interventions for adults and children receiving palliative care: A systematic review. *Palliative Medicine*, *35*(3), pp. 529–551.

Breitbart, W., Poppito, S., Rosenfeld, B., Vickers, A.J., Li, Y., Abbey, J., Olden, M., Pessin, H., Lichtenthal, W., Sjoberg, D. and Cassileth, B.R., 2012. Pilot randomized controlled trial of individual meaning-centered psychotherapy for patients with advanced cancer. *Journal of Clinical Oncology*, *30*(12), p.1304.

Breitbart, W., Rosenfeld, B., Gibson, C., Pessin, H., Poppito, S., Nelson, C., Tomarken, A., Timm, A.K., Berg, A., Jacobson, C. and Sorger, B., 2010. Meaning-centered group psychotherapy for patients with advanced cancer: a pilot randomized controlled trial. *Psycho-Oncology*, *19*(1), pp.21–28.

Breitbart, W., Rosenfeld, B., Pessin, H., Applebaum, A., Kulikowski, J. and Lichtenthal, W.G., 2015. Meaning-centered group psychotherapy: an effective intervention for improving psychological well-being in patients with advanced cancer. *Journal of Clinical Oncology*, *33*(7), p.749.

Breitbart, W., Rosenfeld, B., Pessin, H., Kaim, M., Funesti-Esch, J., Galietta, M., Nelson, C.J. and Brescia, R., 2000. Depression, hopelessness, and desire for hastened death in terminally ill patients with cancer. *JAMA*, *284*(22), pp.2907–2911.

Bruner, M.L., 2002. *Strategies of Remembrance: The Rhetorical Dimensions of National Identity Construction*. Univ of South Carolina Press.

Bunzli, S., Watkins, R., Smith, A., Schütze, R. and O'Sullivan, P., 2013. Lives on hold: a qualitative synthesis exploring the experience of chronic low-back pain. *The Clinical Journal of Pain*, *29*(10), pp.907–916.

Bury, M., 1982. Chronic illness as biographical disruption. *Sociology of Health & Illness*, *4*(2), pp.167–182.

Carroll, E. and Romano, J., 2010. *Your Digital Afterlife: When Facebook, Flickr and Twitter Are Your Estate, What's Your Legacy?* New Riders.

Chiang, K.J., Chu, H., Chang, H.J., Chung, M.H., Chen, C.H., Chiou, H.Y. and Chou, K.R., 2010. The effects of reminiscence therapy on psychological well-being, depression, and loneliness among the institutionalized aged. *International Journal of Geriatric Psychiatry: A journal of the psychiatry of late life and allied sciences*, *25*(4), pp.380–388.

Chochinov, H.M., 2004. Dignity and the eye of the beholder. *Journal of Clinical Oncology*, *22*(7), pp.1336–1340.

Chochinov, H.M., 2012. *Dignity Therapy: Final Words for Final Days*. OUP USA.

Chochinov, H.M., Hack, T., Hassard, T., Kristjanson, L.J., McClement, S. and Harlos, M., 2005. Dignity therapy: a novel psychotherapeutic intervention for patients near the end of life. *J Clin Oncol*, *23*(24), pp.5520–5525.
Chung, H.M., Lyckholm, L.J. and Smith, T.J., 2009. Palliative care in BMT. *Bone Marrow Transplantation*, *43*(4), pp.265–273.
Ciambrone, D.E., 2001. Illness and other assaults on self: the relative impact of HIV/AIDS on women's lives. *Sociology of Health & Illness*, *23*(4), pp.517–540.
Coleman, P., 1999. The legacy of Rousseau, and: Rousseau and the politics of ambiguity, and: the 'confessions' and correspondence, including the letters to Malesherbes. *Eighteenth-Century Studies*, *33*(1), pp.152–153.
Crettaz, B. (2010) Cafés mortels *[Death Cafes]*, Labor et Fides.
Erikson, E.H., 1968. Identity and identity diffusion. *Ch. Gordon and KJ Gergen (Eds.), The Self in Social Interaction. Vol. I: Classic and Contemporary Perspectives, New York (John Wiley & Sons) 1968*, pp. 197–206.
Frankl, V.E., 1947/2021. *Man's Search for Meaning*. Simon and Schuster.
Gibson, C.A. and Breitbart, W., 2004. Individual meaning-centered psychotherapy treatment manual. *Unpublished document.*
Gulotta, R., Odom, W., Forlizzi, J. and Faste, H., 2013, April. Digital artifacts as legacy: exploring the lifespan and value of digital data. In *Proceedings of the SIGCHI Conference on Human Factors in Computing Systems* (pp. 1813–1822).
Haber, D., 2006. Life review: Implementation, theory, research, and therapy. *The International Journal of Aging and Human Development*, *63*(2), pp.153–171.
Heidegger, M., 1962. *Being and Time* (J. Macquarrie and E. Robinson, trans.), Harper and Row.
Hilgeman, M.M., Allen, R.S., Snow, A.L., Durkin, D.W., DeCoster, J. and Burgio, L., 2014. Preserving Identity and Planning for Advance Care (PIPAC): preliminary outcomes from a patient-centered intervention for individuals with mild dementia. *Aging & Mental Health*, *18*(4), pp.411–424.
Hunter, E.G. and Rowles, G.D., 2005. Leaving a legacy: Toward a typology. *Journal of Aging Studies*, *19*(3), pp.327–347.
Hunter, E.G., 2008. The legacy of cancer: The importance of passing on beliefs, values, and positive health behaviors for women with cancer. *Journal of Psychosocial Oncology*, *26*(1), pp.101–121.
Irwin, R.S. and Richardson, N.D., 2006. Patient-focused care: using the right tools. *Chest*, *130*(1), pp.73S–82S.
Julião, M., Antunes, B., Santos, A., Sobral, M.A., Albuquerque, S., Fareleira, F., Runa, D., de Sousa, P.F., Chaves, P., Gonçalves, C. and Soares, D., 2020a. Adapting the Portuguese dignity question framework for adolescents: Ages 10–18. *Palliative & Supportive Care*, *18*(2), pp.199–205.
Julião, M., Santos, A., Albuquerque, S., Antunes, B., Crujo, M., Sobral, M.A., Cancelinha, C., da Silva Soares, D., Fradique, E., Palaré, M.J. and Chochinov, H.M., 2020b. Operationalizing dignity therapy for adolescents. *Palliative & Supportive Care*, *18*(5), pp.626–631.
Kastenbaum, R., 2000. *The Psychology of Death*. Springer Publishing Company.
Kotre, J.N., 1984. Maestro Antonino. *Phenomenology+ Pedagogy*, *2*, pp.136–138.
Lawford, H.L., Astrologo, L., Ramey, H.L. and Linden-Andersen, S., 2020. Identity, intimacy, and generativity in adolescence and young adulthood: A test of the psychosocial model. *Identity*, *20*(1), pp.9–21.
Lazarus, R.S. and Folkman, S., 1984. *Stress, Appraisal, and Coping*. Springer Publishing Company.

Lichtenthal, W.G., Roberts, K.E., Catarozoli, C., Schofield, E., Holland, J.M., Fogarty, J.J., Coats, T.C., Barakat, L.P., Baker, J.N., Brinkman, T.M. and Neimeyer, R.A., 2020. Regret and unfinished business in parents bereaved by cancer: a mixed methods study. *Palliative Medicine*, *34*(3), pp.367–377.

Lloyd-Williams, M., Cobb, M., O'Connor, C., Dunn, L. and Shiels, C., 2013. A pilot randomised controlled trial to reduce suffering and emotional distress in patients with advanced cancer. *Journal of Affective Disorders*, *148*(1), pp.141–145.

Lowton, K., Hiley, C. and Higgs, P., 2017. Constructing embodied identity in a 'new'ageing population: A qualitative study of the pioneer cohort of childhood liver transplant recipients in the UK. *Social Science & Medicine*, *172*, pp.1–9.

Mastel-Smith, B., Binder, B., Malecha, A., Hersch, G., Symes, L. and McFarlane, J., 2006. Testing therapeutic life review offered by home care workers to decrease depression among home-dwelling older women. *Issues in Mental Health Nursing*, *27*(10), pp.1037–1049.

McAdams, D.P., 1987. A life-story model of identity. In *Perspectives in Personality* (pp. 15–50). JAI Press.

McAdams, D.P., 1996. Personality, modernity, and the storied self: A contemporary framework for studying persons. *Psychological inquiry*, 7(4), pp.295–321.

McAdams, D.P., de St Aubin, E.D. and Logan, R.L., 1993. Generativity among young, midlife, and older adults. *Psychology and aging*, *8*(2), p.221.

McClement, S., Chochinov, H.M., Hack, T., Hassard, T., Kristjanson, L.J. and Harlos, M., 2007. Dignity therapy: family member perspectives. *Journal of Palliative Medicine*, *10*(5), pp.1076–1082.

Miles, L. and Corr, C.A., 2017. Death cafe: What is it and what we can learn from it. *OMEGA-Journal of Death and Dying*, *75*(2), pp.151–165.

Monaghan, L.F. and Gabe, J., 2015. Chronic illness as biographical contingency? Young people's experiences of asthma. *Sociology of Health & Illness*, *37*(8), pp.1236–1253.

Monaghan, L.F. and Gabe, J., 2016. Embodying health identities: A study of young people with asthma. *Social Science & Medicine*, *160*, pp.1–8.

Montross, L., Winters, K.D. and Irwin, S.A., 2011. Dignity therapy implementation in a community-based hospice setting. *Journal of Palliative Medicine*, *14*(6), pp.729–734.

Papalia, D.E., Sterns, H.L., Feldman, R.D. and Camp, C.J., 2007. *Adult Development and Aging*. McGraw-Hill.

Perese, E.F., Simon, M.R. and Ryan, E., 2008. Promoting positive student clinical experiences with older adults through use of group reminiscence therapy. *Journal of Gerontological Nursing*, *34*(12), pp.46–51.

Pinquart, M. and Fröhlich, C., 2009. Psychosocial resources and subjective well-being of cancer patients. *Psychology and Health*, *24*(4), pp.407–421.

Ricoeur, P., 1984. Time and Narrative, translated by K. McLaughlin and D. Pellauer. Chicago, University of Chicago Press, *8*, p.160.

Rodin, G. and Gillies, L.A., 2009. Individual psychotherapy for the patient with advanced disease. *Handbook of Psychiatry in Palliative Medicine*. London: Oxford University, pp.443–53.

Rodriguez, A., Smith, J. and McDermid, K., 2018. Dignity therapy interventions for young people in palliative care: a rapid structured evidence review. *International Journal of Palliative Nursing*, *24*(7), pp.339–349.

Sanders, J., 2015. *Adaptation and Appropriation*. Routledge.

Sanderson, T., Calnan, M., Morris, M., Richards, P. and Hewlett, S., 2011. Shifting normalities: interactions of changing conceptions of a normal life and the normalisation of symptoms in rheumatoid arthritis. *Sociology of Health & Illness*, *33*(4), pp.618–633.

Scannell, K.A., 2000. Leave of absence. *Annals of Internal Medicine*, *132*(1), pp.55–57.

Schuelke, T. and Rubenstein, J., 2020. Dignity therapy in pediatrics: A case series. *Palliative Medicine Reports*, *1*(1), pp.156–160.

Sherman, D.W., Norman, R. and McSherry, C.B., 2010. A comparison of death anxiety and quality of life of patients with advanced cancer or AIDS and their family caregivers. *Journal of the Association of Nurses in AIDS Care*, *21*(2), pp.99–112.

Skeath, P., Norris, S., Katheria, V., White, J., Baker, K., Handel, D., Sternberg, E., Pollack, J., Groninger, H., Phillips, J. and Berger, A., 2013. The nature of life-transforming changes among cancer survivors. *Qualitative Health Research*, *23*(9), pp.1155–1167.

Sofka, C., 2020. The transition from life to the digital afterlife: Thanatechnology and its impact on grief. In *Digital Afterlife* (pp. 57–74). Chapman and Hall/CRC.

Spitznagel, M.B., Tremont, G., Davis, J.D. and Foster, S.M., 2006. Psychosocial predictors of dementia caregiver desire to institutionalize: caregiver, care recipient, and family relationship factors. *Journal of Geriatric Psychiatry and Neurology*, *19*(1), pp.16–20.

Steger, M.F., Frazier, P., Oishi, S. and Kaler, M., 2006. The meaning in life questionnaire: assessing the presence of and search for meaning in life. *Journal of Counseling Psychology*, *53*(1), p.80.

Steinhauser, K.E., Alexander, S.C., Byock, I.R., George, L.K., Olsen, M.K. and Tulsky, J.A., 2008. Do preparation and life completion discussions improve functioning and quality of life in seriously ill patients? Pilot randomized control trial. *Journal of Palliative Medicine*, *11*(9), pp.1234–1240.

Swaab, D.F., Dubelaar, E.J.G., Hofman, M.A., Scherder, E.J.A., Van Someren, E.J.W. and Verwer, R.W.H., 2002. Brain aging and Alzheimer's disease; use it or lose it. *Progress in Brain Research*, *138*, pp.343–373.

Van Manen, M., 1990. Beyond assumptions: Shifting the limits of action research. *Theory into Practice*, *29*(3), pp.152–157.

Waltman, M.A., Russell, D.C., Coyle, C.T., Enright, R.D., Holter, A.C. and M. Swoboda, C., 2009. The effects of a forgiveness intervention on patients with coronary artery disease. *Psychology and Health*, *24*(1), pp.11–27.

Watts, L., Rodriguez, A., Tatterton, M., McSherry, W. and Smith, J., 2019. Meaning making and Generativity in children and young people with life limiting conditions (MAGICYL). *Evidence-Based Nursing*, *22*, 33–35.

Watts, L., Smith, J., McSherry, W., Tatterton, M. and Rodriguez, A., 2020a. Stakeholder perceptions of dignity therapy for children and young people with life-limiting and life-threatening conditions in the UK. *OBM Integrative and Complementary Medicine*, *5*(1), pp.1–1.

Watts, L., Smith, J., McSherry, W., Tatterton, M. and Rodriguez, A., 2020b. Correction: Watts L, et al. *Stakeholder Perceptions of Dignity Therapy for Children and Young People with Life-Limiting and Life-Threatening Conditions in the UK*. OBM Integrative and Complementary Medicine.

Williams, S., 2000. Chronic illness as biographical disruption or biographical disruption as chronic illness? Reflections on a core concept. *Sociology of Health & Illness*, *22*(1), pp.40–67.

Yalom, I.D., 1980/2020. *Existential Psychotherapy*. Hachette UK.

6 The lived experience of serious illness

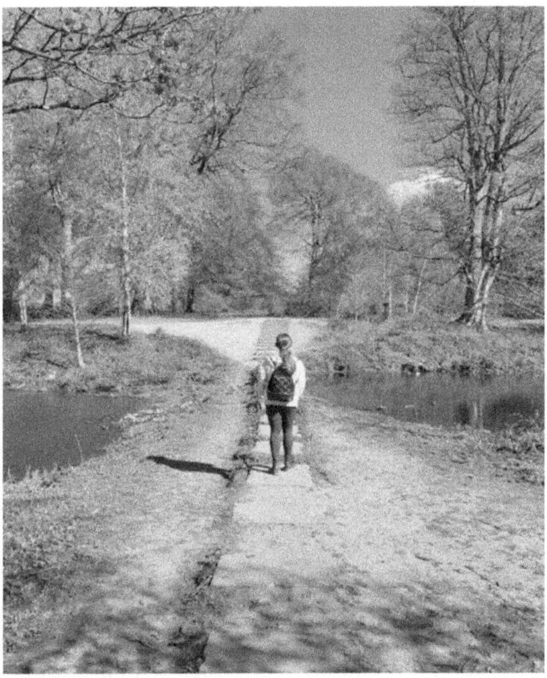

Figure 6.1 A photograph of a person walking on a dirt path. Photograph taken by Alison Rodriguez.

Introduction

To live is our human pursuit, dying although inevitable, is something we do not invest much of our attention in (Bauman, 1992). Over the last thirty years we have however, embraced a new medical age, appreciating the multi-dimensional nature of health and illness. The health and illness evidence base,

DOI: 10.4324/9781003340287-7

from the perspective of health and social care professionals now also commonly refers to the 'journey' metaphor to illuminate individual's lived experiences from health to illness, from diagnosis to recovery or indeed to death (Hvidt, 2017). The 'illness journey' takes its travellers or 'patients' via different routes to their destinations. One such route is medically driven, scooping up all available treatments for cure. Other routes extend beyond biomedicine, unveiling the emotionality of the experience. Each traveller possesses unique psycho-social, existential, and spiritual qualities that enable their passage. At times, the traveller will wonder off track and need support to access, manage and build on these qualities. Although pain and sadness can sometimes prevail, there remains scope for wellbeing, personal growth, and transformation.

On receipt of a life threatening or life limiting diagnosis, individuals and/or families face their first blip in their journey. The life journey they had planned takes a new course and further changes are ahead, not just with respect to future horizons and planned for events, but with everyday living. The road ahead is a challenge, laybys need to be in sight to take on board the treatments and to reflect on those parts of life that hold the most meaning. Relationships and ways of being change and the individual may need time to be able to accommodate these changes that affect themselves and significant others in their lives.

According to Husserl, the founding father of phenomenology (1983: 124), individuals engage with a phenomenological mission throughout their lived experiences. Playing close attention to their lived experiences their challenge is to be conscious of, perceive and remember the multiple phenomena in their lifeworld's (Lebenswelt). The Lebenswelt for Husserl is our shared world of meanings, experiences, and pre-judgments, relevant to each context in which we are situated. We take for granted our everyday worlds, that we co-habit with our 'home fellows' (Heimgenossen). This everyday world however is sanctioned when individuals are moved into the alien world of life limitedness, which with time establishes a level of familiarity and normality for those within it (Steinbock, 1995: 187).

Individuals, families and carers strive to achieve a normality; however, they are thrown into a world out of touch with their everyday world. Entering an alien or unready world can be likened in keeping with the journey metaphor, to embarking upon an adventure; the endpoint of which is both mobile and invisible. The journey is not determined but instead unfolds, allowing the future to slowly reveal itself as it releases the present (Heidegger, 1996). Faircloth et al. (2004) described how some individuals engage in a continuous life narrative that integrates their illness experiences: a process they called biographical flow. This biographical flow has a depth of meaning, identifying disruption to assumptions about the world and how things, events and the self are perceived. Accordingly, a continuous self-narrative allows emotional wellbeing, when there is a biographical disruption, then occurs emotional disruption also (Bury, 1982; Giddens, 1991). Illness itself can be a disruption, but if the self-narrative can accommodate it then there are limited threats to identity. This biographical account of illness reflects contemporary notions of the self as a 'reflexive project' through lived experiences (Giddens, 1991: 75). (See also the biographical disruption section of Chapter 5).

Liminality and embodiment

'Liminality' has evolved from the Latin word 'limen' which translates to 'threshold' in English. A threshold is the divide that is created by a door opening and one that we pass through to move from one room to another. The journey of a life threatening/limiting condition is fraught with challenging times and places that individuals and their significant others must cross through – the threshold or liminality is the unbounded space that is created by those challenges. These liminal spaces are uncomfortable, they can be long and enduring. The concept of liminality, however, provides the individual and their significant others with some recognition of that place that can feel very much like a 'no man's land', a place to dwell with the more existential and spiritual aspects of the self, of time and of meaning and purpose. For example, the individual will reflect on their life before illness, or situated between crises, teetering on the edge of further degeneration, they may ruminate on the characteristics of their illness and what further uncertain periods they may have in front of them, what further liminal spaces may lie ahead.

It is the palliative care team who embrace their expertise in times like this, supporting and being present with individuals and families. For example, the palliative care nurse will walk with the individual and family and more closely at these junctures; the chaplain who will support spiritual movement; the psychologist who will help guide adjustment processes, or the advanced nurse specialist or medical doctor who will try their best to ease the physical symptoms of pain and anguish. The team stand strong within and thereafter these liminal times and spaces (Cohen-Gogo et al., 2011).

When caring for children and young people with palliative care needs, teams can have a more complex task, needing to accommodate the liminal spaces that are as much defined by developmental stage and cognitive abilities of the individual as by their disease and its stage of progression. Perceptions of normative life orders are thrown into jeopardy and children and young people can be left wondering not just about their own existence and futures but what the role of illness and family means to their lifetimes too. Parents are often overburdened with having to assist with cares and to shoulder the emotion of the now and the future, each with different coping styles, each wanting more understanding to help them negotiate the whys. Instrumental support for parents is paramount to enable child, young person, and family to travel this journey, professionals must juggle these liminal spaces by drawing on their experience and in doing so balance parental hope against reality (Rodriguez, 2009).

How we understand and conceptualise these experiences and liminal spaces is subjective and embodied, we do not just exist and experience, we feel and experience (Williams and Bendelow, 1998). Charmaz (2002) has argued that we can over narrate experiences, focusing down on the words people use to express themselves. However, we should also be exploring the moments of silence and consider the importance of what is not said which can be equivocal or more informative than looking over what is said. This can be especially relevant to the field of palliative care. Not all individuals can communicate verbally, and people reach points in their illnesses whereby they can no longer speak or communicate effectively with others using verbal communication. If we take the example of individuals with neuro degenerative conditions, if we constructed notions of self only as derived from language then we may fail to reach these individuals and the worth of their emotions in understanding their illness experiences (Sabat et al., 1999).

Merleau-Ponty (1968) argued that Being is a bodily experience, we bodily react and reciprocate to our environments and experiences. It is in this way that our experiences are framed by our perceptions of them. The phenomenological understanding of this is 'being part of the world' (Merleau-Ponty, 1962).

Suffering and total pain

Dame Cicely Saunders, the person who influenced the modern hospice movement, would refer to the term 'total pain'. Total pain is an example of our embodied being in the world, an all-encompassing experience of body and mind (Kleinman, 1997). This also illustrates how pain itself can be liminal. Pain frequently accompanies the palliative care experience for individuals (Downey et al., 2009) and can be physical (e.g., intractable pain), psychological (e.g., anxiety, depression, hopelessness), religious (e.g., crisis of faith), or social (e.g., disintegration of human relationships). Spiritual pain is the culmination of a few or all these aspects and can be manifested externally in characteristic behaviours displayed by individuals. For example, there are individuals who express clear desperation to escape their lived realities; individuals who pose unrealistic demands/challenges for their main care givers; individuals who continue to search for cure despite there being no real hope of one; individuals who demand increasing pain relief to no benefit. Such behaviours can also be classified as expressions of suffering, but such can lead us also to the nature of the pain.

The International Association for the Study of Pain (IASP) (2022) defines pain as *'an unpleasant sensory and emotional experience associated with actual or potential tissue damage'*. In addition, if the individual cannot communicate verbally, it is acknowledged that this does not mean they are not suffering pain. As such we can appreciate that the notion of 'total pain' is congruent with 'mainstream' pain theory.

The gate control theory of pain details how the expression and experience of pain is often initiated or calibrated even by emotion and cognitive perception (Melzack and Wall, 1965). Indeed, it is conceptualized that pain is a perceptual and affective experience influenced by the individual's levels of attention, anxiety, and other psychological variables such as past experiences, ascribed meanings of pain, current emotionality and in what ways sensory nerve patterns are activated by physical stimulation (Melzack, 1982). To understand the subjective experience of pain we therefore need to explore the unique experience of the individual and not just try to delineate potential root (and often focus on physical) causes.

Pain should also be evaluated with respect to its effect on family members and carers. Relational issues can intensify the pain experience and therefore it is appropriate that a definition considers the importance of relationality in pain expression and experience. Often the struggles individuals have at the end of life relate to leaving their loved ones behind, in searching for meaning around this and their demise, the individual can struggle with their faith and in hinging on any meaning or purpose and this can also exacerbate the pain experience (Downing and Luyirika, 2018).

Unrelieved pain

There is a consensus that to not have pain resolved risks individual dignity (Periyakoil et al., 2009). Historically, there was more attention paid to adult pain as it was understood that children did not experience pain as heightened as adult do. Research however has identified that children and adults can experience similar levels of pain intensity (Anand et al., 1997). For parents, to see a child in pain or to perceive they have pain is difficult, a worst case scenario is when pain cannot be eliminated.

In practice, much reliance is paid upon self-report of pain, especially in older children and adults. The determination of pain and levels of pain in younger children however is more complex, not just relating to age and level of vocabulary but developmental understanding of what pain is and how to express their discomfort to communicate needs. Where possible it is advocated therefore that professionals use childlike language to be able to enter the world of the child and engage their expression of and severity of the pain and its origin. It is also important to note that any questioning about pain may be responded to differently by the child as they will attach meaning and implication to their answers. If the child is fearful of medical intervention for example, then they may fear discussing their pain with professionals in the mind that such could result in invasive procedures.

Without verbal communication willingness or ability, professionals can use their observation skills. Expression of discomfort in acute pain differs to more chronic and enduring pain in children. With acute pain children can be active and noisy, whereas with more chronic pain there can be a withdrawal, a lack of interest, sleeping disturbance and clinginess with parents (Chambers et al., 1998). Discussions with parents are also valuable but they sometimes can underestimate pain levels. Vital signs can alter but heart rate and pulse can also indicate fear – and even though child pain measures are evolving around acute pain, there is difficultly in using such and considering their reliability for potential chronic pain cases. Like with adults, past experiences, and an understanding of the child's pain threshold, how pain is considered and expressed by the family and the child's emotional state, are all useful factors to be aware of in interpreting the pain of a child.

Many adult centric scales exist for the purpose of self-report pain assessment and measurement, but these are often not of any use to young people with neuro degeneration because there may for example be a reliance on memory – has your pain improved? For example, and can you identify the main site of the pain? Such tools also require a proficient level of verbal articulation. As some conditions progress memory and verbal ability decreases which can render pain assessment and management to be of a similar standing of such in very young children. Recently, however the Mobilization-Observation-Behavior-Intensity-Dementia-2 (MOBID-2) Pain Scale (Husebo et al., 2007), a purely observational tool, has shown good levels of reliability for individuals with advanced dementia and therefore may also have utility for young people with neurodegenerative conditions.

As already briefly noted, the cultural norms of the family about pain perception are also important, similarly the wider cultural norms relevant to individuals and families are important. Evidence to date however is not consistent regarding race and ethnicity and pain expression, assessment and management. Some studies argue there are no disparities, whilst others suggest that white individuals report more frequently their pain and anxiety (Muni et al., 2011). When looking specifically at individuals within end of life care it has been found that regardless of cultural heritage, most individuals benefit from hospice and palliative care with equivocal pain and symptom management. What is of interest however is the fact that individuals from minority ethnic backgrounds are less likely to accept hospice and palliative care provision at the end of their life (Boucher and Johnson, 2021). A number of authors have highlighted the reported difficulties. They include a perception that the racial and religious disparity between carers and individuals will leave needs unmet (Yancu et al., 2010). As such, the complexity of treating individuals with 'total pain' is often compounded by the individuals' inability to see the worth in palliative and related hospice care provision, alongside their ability to both determine and describe their pain to their family/carers and indeed their willingness to do so.

Lived experiences and quality of life

Like pain, the concept of a good quality of life (QOL) is hard to define but holds some meaning for us all. Theoretically is has been defined as having a number of parts or aspects to it that impact on global life satisfaction, incorporating good health, housing, employment, safety, interrelationships, education, and leisure activities. In terms of exploring QOL as specifically relevant to a health condition or care, the term 'health-related quality of life' (HRQL) has been coined (Bergner, 1989).

The concept of HRQL, explores life quality as affected by health status, therefore considers the impact of disease symptomology, treatment effects and satisfaction, physical and psycho-social functioning and wellbeing, emotional and cognitive health, in its evaluation. A number of measures have evolved from more mainstream health psychology practice with individuals with chronic disease or long term conditions. Length of survival was once considered a most important factor for quality of life, whereas now the impacts of illness are more closely and importantly considered (Kluetz et al., 2016).

HRQL has been a central issue for cancer care for some time.

Karnofsky and Burchenal (1949) introduced a clinical scale to quantify the functional performance of individuals with cancer (Schag et al., 1984). This increased professional interest in the assessment of HRQL and influenced the further development of standardized, self-administered measures. HRQOL has also become a key focus for more novel treatments and therapies.

HRQL is viewed to be of significance to individuals in the later stages of their illnesses. Indeed, palliative care, focused on relieving pain and suffering, also aims to achieve the best QOL for individuals and families as possible. Through the duration of physical illness individuals will experience comorbid psychological difficulties (Griffin and Fentiman, 2002). Both physical and mental health issues can compromise QOL. It is imperative that professionals keep a check on the emotional and psychological wellbeing of individuals as poor mental health can exacerbate the physical condition. Assessment and evaluation of day-to-day activities can provide an insight into how the individual is coping. For some individuals, the fatigue and pain of their conditions can render them socially isolated. This and other psychosocial factor (e.g., stigma of illness, lack of support, and perceived illness intrusiveness) can influence an individual's quality of life in many ways. For example, low mood, difficult relationship issues, lower sense of wellbeing and heightened emotional distress. If these issues go unnoticed then life threatening/limiting conditions can increasingly cause suffering, distress, anxiety, and depression (Weis and Boehncke, 2011).

Quality of life outcomes can be related to fear and uncertainty. In addition, the reaction to changes or to prognosis can cause a number of psychosocial effects that impact on the personal and social world views. Although over the years we have borne witness to much medical and technological advances, there has been sparse attention placed on helping individuals manage the psychosocial demands and impacts of their condition on their QOL (Fann et al., 2012).

Although individuals with palliative care needs experience many changes, the feeling of a loss of 'self' is all encompassing and can impact on several psychosocial outcomes associated with low levels of control, feelings of worthlessness, autonomy, and increased dependency (Nilmanat et al. 2010). This is reported with particularly high prevalence in studies of individuals aged 25–40 years old. The disruption of life threatening/limiting illness can influence an individuals need to control every other aspect of their lives until death, because everything else feels so much out of their control (Volker and Wu, 2011).

Where there is no hope for a cure it could be presumed that the individual is left to feel hopeless. Several studies however have identified that it is only a small subset of the end-of-life population who are unable to relieve any sense of hopelessness. These individuals are often also suffering from comorbid depression and can be fixated on a hastened death (Parpa et al., 2019; van Laarhoven et al., 2011). The noted relationship between hopelessness and suicidal thoughts evokes an understanding of how difficult life can be for those facing death. Individuals who report increased psychospiritual well-being, however, appear to cope better and are able to find some reason for their experience. Familial and social support, prognostic knowledge and autonomy are also factors considered to support individual's status. Whereas emotional distress, anxiety, helplessness, hopelessness and fear of death diminishes wellbeing, feeling a burden to others can also be an overwhelming feeling for young people, and impact on quality-of-life outcomes (Cohen and Leis, 2002). Self-perceived burden is defined as

> *a multidimensional construct arising from the care-recipient's feelings of dependence and the resulting frustration and worry, which then lead to negative feelings of guilt at being responsible for the caregiver's hardship.*
>
> (Cousineau et al., 2003, p.111)

Among individuals with serious illness, sensing oneself as a burden to others seems to be an important theme related to quality of life, optimal palliative care, and maintenance of dignity at the end of life (Cohen and Leis, 2002). Indeed, most health and social care professionals would argue that a large focus of their cares are to enhance QOL outcomes, and that individual dignity is central to care delivery. Chochinov (2002) as briefly mentioned in Chapter 5, developed a model of dignity conserving care. The model details what factors can enhance or support dignity as individuals live through their serious illnesses. This model has also been used as the basis of psychotherapeutic intervention and contains three categories of dignity care:

1. Attention to illness-related issues pertaining to bodily concerns or problems.
2. The adoption of a dignity-conserving repertoire which addresses the individuals psychological and spiritual beliefs; and
3. A social dignity inventory, referring to external influences affecting dignity (Chochinov et al., 2002, p.2255).

Illness-related concerns are issues that are illness specific, relevant to symptomology and physical strains on the individual's ability for example their ability to maintain self-cares and other activities that would require levels of independence to conduct or complete. By independence this can relate to both physical ability and mental acuity.

The *dignity-conserving repertoire* is spilt in two parts: 'dignity-conserving perspectives' and 'dignity-conserving practices'. Perspectives can be related to:

- Continuity of self
- Role preservation
- Generativity/legacy

- Maintaining pride
- Maintaining hope
- Autonomy/control
- Acceptance
- Resilience/fighting spirit.

Dignity-conserving practices involve a 'living in the moment', rather than thinking too far ahead into the future. Maintaining routine whilst seeking to cope with physical and emotional now challenges of illness and seeking spiritual comfort.

The *social dignity inventory* is about the quality of interactions with others and how such can enhance a feeling of dignity. There are five external sources of dignity enhancement within this domain:

- Privacy boundaries: dignity can be affected by others entering their care receiving spaces
- Social support: helpful others
- Care tenor: the attitude (empathy/compassion) of others who care
- Burden to others: relying on others can be overbearing
- Aftermath concerns: concern for the burden their death may bring about for their significant others.

This model of dignity has been described by Chochinov as a 'therapeutic map' that can assist professionals to observe for difficulties and to provide support where needed. Bearing witness, validating concerns and assisting meaning making can also increase dignity at the end of our lives (Chochinov et al., 2004).

Instrumental support

Instrumental support refers to support that is practical; help that means tasks can be completed, for example help with chores or attending clinics. This type of support is corelated with increased wellbeing outcomes.

Loss of identity or of significant roles is related to existential suffering. Helping individuals to appreciate that there are still many aspects of life unaffected by their condition is of therapeutic value. For example, a mother feeling she is no longer acting as a parent to all her children because so much of her time is devoted to the sick child can find benefit in being told that her other children are gaining useful insight into how to deal with a difficult experience. Some parents facing their own death also like to create legacy projects for their children so that they can feel some parental presence and active support through their lives. Parents will worry about the burden of care they are placing on their children and sometimes can be upset by the magnitude of the role reversal. This can be resultant of the parent themselves being in receipt of palliative care or the parent being reliant on dependent children to help with the cares of a sibling with serious illness.

Children with serious illness are a unique population. We often talk to children about what they would like to be when they grow up. This is one drastic change of Being, if your child is not expected to live through to adulthood and for children and young people, they can lose self-worth knowing they are not going to achieve purposeful employment as an adult. It is important that children's existential concerns are not neglected and that professionals actively address these concerns, of course also being mindful of the child's developmental stage (Hoffmaster, 2011; Bates and Kearney, 2015).

Supporting family members

A priority focus of palliative care is supporting the many family and lay caregivers who care and support individuals with serious illness. The stress that can be involved in this role due to the many tasks they must undertake for individuals and often with no or very little training, can lead to high rates of anxiety, depression, and poor quality of life (Geng et al., 2018), lowered attention to self-care and increased risk of heart problems (Nicholas Dionne-Odom et al., 2017). With women more involved in direct caring roles, the prevalence of these negative events is higher within this gender group (Bom and Stöckel, 2021)). As more children are born with palliative care needs, more children are living longer with serious illness, more young people are transitioning to adult services and the benefits of familial care are recognised to save financial burden on formal care services, it is likely that the instrumental support demands on family carers will increase in the years to come. Therefore, health and social care professionals, in being providers of family centred care in the context of palliative care, also need to look out for the support needs of carers, to reduce shared distress and to help relief carer burden.

Providing support to both individuals with serious illness and their families is written in practice guidelines. Instrumental social support, by definition, provides practical and emotional resources to others to assist them to cope with stressful life events. Theoretically, instrumental support that assists care givers with their giving tasks can also support their coping with the situation (Nishio et al., 2017). However, there remains a lack of population-based studies that explore the impact of formal instrumental support provided to family caregivers. The evidence base however, is replete with studies that identify carer burden and support needs (Rodriguez and King, 2009; Rodriguez and King, 2014).

Adjusting boundaries

Health and social care professionals offer emotional support to individuals and families by establishing a therapeutic relationship. Where boundaries are overstepped, this is usually considered to be when professionals get over involved with the holistic needs of individuals and families and they offer support outside of their professional identity, or when the support offered is beyond that expected. This can lead to professionals becoming too emotionally close to individuals or over attached (Roberts et al., 2015).

There are studies however that have identified that due to the very nature of palliative care, there can be times where boundaries become a little blurred (Reid, 2013). Where health and social care professionals are caring for the seriously ill and dying there is a need for a more personal and emotional involvement in role.

In studies of nurses supporting seriously ill children for example, there have been reports of them reflecting on their own beliefs and values about death and dying (Keenan and Mac Dermott, 2016; Reid, 2013) and discussion of how nurses will often have responded to individuals' deaths with grief, sadness, hurting, moral distress, struggling and suffering.

Joshua Wales, a physician wrote a blog recently in the *New England Journal of Medicine* (a USA based international periodical), reflecting on how easily boundaries can be adjusted in palliative care to help ease the suffering of individuals and to support their personhood:

> *'You must sing for me', she said. 'I'm dying, after all'. Ms. N. was sitting on her vast white sofa, frail among the cushions, enveloped in a pink dressing gown that paled next to the fuchsia of her lipstick. She was partially silhouetted by the late November sun from the wall of windows behind her. In her right hand, she held a flute of champagne, and she closed her eyes as she sipped from it. Her malignant bowel obstruction made swallowing impossible, however, so she spat the champagne into a glass bowl beside her. I smiled and looked at the floor, trying to will the request away. We had met earlier in the week during my first visit as her home palliative care physician, and I was getting used to the brusque cadence of her Eastern European accent, just as she was no doubt getting used to my questions about her pain and nausea. Today, however, the tables had turned abruptly: in a conversation about her extensive record collection, my other career as an opera singer had surfaced. This aspect of my life became the focus of her line of questions. 'I'm not sure that singing is such a good idea', I said, trying to reorient the spotlight. This visit wasn't about me, after all; it was about her. I was keen to occupy as little space as possible. 'But you must', she insisted. I had never sung for a patient before, and the thought of it was odd and uncomfortable. In asking me to sing, she was asking me to cross a boundary – that invisible line in medicine that marks the edges of professional behaviour appropriate to our clinical roles (*Chen et al., 2018*). We learn in medical school to maintain a distance between ourselves and our patients. We hide any parts of our personal histories that risk distracting from the patient's narrative. First and foremost, we represent the profession of medicine. Our individuality takes a back seat (*Curran, 2014; Lussier et al., 2007*) Indeed, there is a kind of safety in the distance created by the well-defined roles of patient and physician. Boundary crossings create uncertainty – we move away from a clearly demarcated clinical relationship to something much more nebulous and potentially destabilizing for both parties. (*Lussier et al., 2007*) We also risk shifting the focus from the patient to the physician; a physician's disclosure of personal information to a patient is often more*

> *disruptive than beneficial (*McDonald et al., 2007*). Finally, personal relationships may cloud both our judgment and that of our patients. But at the same time, patients want physicians who aren't robots, who are friendly and relatable. Is there a safe way to show patients that we are human while also remaining professional?*
>
> (Wales, 2019, *P1894)*

Helping individuals to find a silver lining

While many impacts of serious illness are deemed negative, there can be times where individuals reach a different worldview and can reflect on the subjective changes that have occurred, things that happened that have made their lives better. Illness of this nature can influence personal growth.

Fletcher (2011) explored the experiences of mothers whose children were receiving care for their cancer conditions or who had recently died. All these women discussed 'silver linings' and mused about how their outlook on life had altered through their experiences. They had made different life priorities and had become more focused on the positive parts of their life, for example (Fletcher, 2011, pp50–51):

> *'I call it my gift of, of appreciating life… So, the sky is a little bluer and the jokes are a little funnier and you just appreciate just that much more. You think about it, you do think about and that's not a bad thing, it's a good thing. It's a really good thing. ~M5'*
>
> *'The other positive I guess would be that I don't plan anymore and I, I'm a lot easier to get along with (chuckle). You know my house always had to be perfect before anybody came over and with [son's name] sick I mean people were coming and going all the time so I couldn't do that. So, it doesn't matter. Its little stuff like that I think I'm trying to look at as positive. ~ M1*
>
> *The cancer experience that [my son] and our family went through was not something that I would ever wish upon anyone, but at the same time a lot of good also came out of it. ~M8*
>
> *I try to find the good in every little thing. I've become more positive. I think I've always been a fairly positive person, but I've become more positive through it all ~M3*
>
> *You learn to look for rainbows in any bad situation and try to remain positive no matter what. You learn to accept things you cannot change, change the things you can, and know the difference. You learn not to sweat the small stuff. ~M6*
>
> *I am not walking through life with blinders on. I thank God for every second I get to spend with my child. ~M9*

Where children had died, mothers had tried their best to make the most of time left:

> *Definitely um, there were a lot of positives. I, um. (pause) I think I did more quality time with my son than I would have if he wasn't ill. So, I have so many special*

memories of things that if he wasn't sick, I don't know that we would have gone as far to do. And I'm hoping that I carry that forward with my daughter you know and just do it because I have such gratification for doing it or having done it that I'm hoping that I continue that. So that's awesome.

The more I was a part of the better. I felt that I was doing all I could do. I, I was very much one of, um, I don't want to have any regrets of not being somewhere, not doing as much as I could have. Well maybe I could have done this or so my big coping that was just being there and, and, um, ya doing, doing whatever it is I could do.

Mothers also reflected on the value of family support and how the experience of palliative care makes you realise how important all family members are:

We don't look at life the same way. [My husband] and I, I think the kids still do, um, but with regards to friends and family I mean you obviously put importance on those things a little bit differently when something like this happens. ~M1

He taught me true love and he taught me, you know, not to stress over the little things. Too fill your life with the people you love the most and the things that mean the most to you. ~M3

Post traumatic growth

Serious illness is regarded as a potential traumatic stressor. Being given a life-threatening or life-limiting diagnosis, enduring pain and intensive treatment and side-effects coupled with an awareness of a shortened life trajectory are together experiences that are 'life-altering' and can severely impact individual's identities, beliefs, and values (Tedeschi et al., 2018).

However, the experience of serious illness and caring for someone with a serious illness, can also lead to transformational change, not least because there have been so many struggles to surmount. Where positive psychological changes are observed, this is viewed as posttraumatic growth (PTG). Individuals change psychologically because of how they have needed to engage personal strength, they have had to change the ways they relate to others, be open to different outcomes in life and develop more of an appreciation for life and spiritual concerns. The Posttraumatic Growth Inventory (PTGI) indicates that growth is an important process for people with serious illness to maintain well-being (Bluvstein et al. 2013).

PTG is regarded as a psychological process that involves a positive cognitive reframing and emotional transformation, resultant of individuals assigning deeper meaning to life events and gaining greater appreciation of life yet to be lived. This process involves a rebuilding of a broken self, a self that has needed to confront life events that have been shattering, that have enforced them to reinvent or reposition themselves through a depth of self-reflection. The lived experience of palliative care emerges as particularly relevant to PTG.

Health and social care professional resilience

Zanatta et al. (2020) recently undertook a systematic review exploring resiliency (successful adaption to and protection from significant stressors) in palliative care professionals. Resilience was significantly correlated with 'professionals experience of death anxiety', 'secondary traumatic stress', 'vicarious post-traumatic growth', 'burnout', 'stress', 'attention to feelings', 'self-esteem', and 'hope'.

The nature of the working environments means that there is regular contact with trauma, with death and dying and suffering. This can lead to professionals experiencing secondary traumatic stress. This will affect their own psychological functioning, but can also influence positive changes in self-perception, interpersonal relationships, and life philosophies. This effect is otherwise labelled vicarious posttraumatic growth. Few studies have explored resilience assessment among palliative care professionals. However, there is a contemporary interest in developing supportive interventions to promote professionals' wellbeing and resilience. The review suggests that resilience can ensue following a meaning construction process that enables professionals to adapt to situations they find themselves in. The ability to cognitively ascribe meaning to stressful situations seems to both enable and maintain resiliency.

Palliative care in situations of crisis

In recent years, there has been more research attention on palliative care provision provided by humanitarian health professionals or the impact on services in times of humanitarian crisis. Authors have situated how important palliative care is when in times of natural disasters, epidemics and war (Smith and Aloudat, 2017). The effective introduction of palliative care in emergency units or intensive care units necessitates tailored training. There are also logistic issues that include protocols of care and individual selection processes that again require specialist knowledge.

Humanitarian crises, like serious illness are a shared experience of emotional and physical burden, accompanied by a fear of death and dying. The availability of care however can be impacted due to movement restrictions. There is often also a restriction on the movement of goods so healthcare resources and treatments become in limited supply. Goals for dignity in care may need to be partially abandoned as palliative care in times of humanitarian crises is fraught with personal and infrastructural difficulties. There is however a dearth of studies that have been able to explore palliative care in these times and the impact on individuals and families lived experiences. There is also research to be done around those who transfer to other countries for safety with serious illness and then become refugees in receipt of palliative care (Cherny, 2007).

Palliative care in times of humanitarian crises can only be improved with specialist training provided to all health and social care providers in anticipation.

However, through the experience of the global pandemic of COVID-19, there are perhaps lessons we can learn for other situations of crisis.

The COVID-19 pandemic

In March 2020, the World Health Organisation declared Coronavirus (COVID-19) a global pandemic (Adams and Walls, 2020). Worldwide, specialist palliative care services have had a valuable role to play in responding to the pandemic, sharing how to provide person-centred symptom control and supported decision making when there remained an elevated level of uncertainty. Where possible advanced care planning needed to be undertaken with individuals and families for both COVID-19 and non-COVID-19 'patients' (and their families). As service organisation altered and visiting restrictions were applied, this did mean that communication was hindered and there was a move to discussing issues with colleagues and families virtually. This situation was compounded by the sheer volume of people being admitted to hospital settings which led to health care professionals less experienced in challenging conversations having to engage in them (van Mol et al., 2022).

In the COVID-19 pandemic it is possible that early intervention from professionals with palliative care experience could have helped communication processes and possibly avoided the prolonged dying processes of some individuals. Many who were supported in intensive care had truly little chance of survival, and yet their final days and weeks of life were mechanically supported in hospital and away from their families.

Palliative care 'patients' with COVID-19

The strict visiting policies and fears of contagion meant providing care and support for individuals dying with COVID-19 was difficult. Caregivers were emotionally impacted by the sheer isolation of end-of-life care, especially at the height of the pandemic. Dying with dignity usually involves the attendance of family wherever possible, and this is of paramount concern to be orchestrated by health and social care professionals. Unfortunately, this was not achieved for many who died of COVID-19. For others, the emotional burden or fear that one would die alone and for caregivers that they would not be present, was traumatic. For these reasons, some hospitals offered virtual visits via electronic devices, these had been quickly provided to various areas of the healthcare system. In good palliative care, frequent and compassionate communication is had between the palliative care team, individuals, and families. However, because of the unpredictable disease trajectory of COVID-19, these communication processes were further hindered. Sometimes communication tasks were also given to unskilled staff. Given the level of complexity, health care professionals who are unfamiliar with palliative care should not be involved. However, the emergency nature and volume of need did necessitate out of the norm processes of care (Sese et al., 2020).

Palliative care for non-COVID-19 'patients'

Palliative care delivery care was impacted by the pandemic. There was (and for many still is) lots of anxiety around both spreading and contracting COVID-19. This made individuals with serious illness hesitant to attend palliative care services and especially hospital settings, and more so once wards were becoming filled with individuals extremely sick with COVID-19.

The COVID-19 crisis impacted patterns of admissions and discharge for individuals with palliative care needs, both within specialised units and hospice care. In the UK, approximately 30% of COVID-19 deaths occurred in care homes (Office for National Statistics, 2020/2021), not least because hospitals were being advised to discharge COVID positive elderly individuals back to their care homes due to ward capacity issues. Strict visit restrictions were applied in hospitals and care homes. Although individuals admitted to acute palliative care units are usually discharged home, those admitted to hospice can have a high mortality rate. This meant caregivers were then very anxious and were found to be saying their goodbyes to individuals on admission. There was also a decrease in hospice admissions in the lockdown period, with families wanting where possible to keep their loved ones at home. There has remained a hesitancy for individuals with serious illness in accessing inpatient care for some time. In more recent months, caregivers in the UK have been permitted to stay with loved ones in the hospice setting but only following proof of their covid free status, following swab testing. There remains a requirement for carers and professionals to be masked (Mercadante, et al., 2020).

Health and social care has been impacted by austerity measures for some time (Marmot et al., 2020). COVID-19 however, further exposed the underfunding and understaffing of services. There were many health and social care professionals struggling with emotional and physical fatigue. In consideration of the increased numbers of healthcare professionals involved in end-of-life care throughout the height of COVID-19 pandemic, several supportive resources such as dedicated education modules have been created to support staff, especially team members less experienced in palliative and end of life direct cares and communication. This is necessary as we realise that COVID-19 is still prevalent with the potential for further mutations in the future (Royal College of Nursing, 2021). The one positive outcome of COVID-19 is that it has highlighted the benefits of peer and team support and how in times of crises whole communities will come together (Maben and Bridges, 2020).

The increased reliance on digital health technology and its impact on palliative care provision

The use of digital technology across services has increased in the wake of the COVID-19 pandemic. A large amount of face-to-face consultations with health and social care professionals for children and young people with palliative care needs have moved to online appointments and interactions. There has also been increased attention given to the development of digital health interventions to assist individuals and families to manage their self-care. Digital health interventions can provide information, support and therapy (for physical, emotional, behavioural and cognitive needs) via an online or digital platform (for example through a website, computer interface, mobile phone application (app), SMS, email, videoconferencing, or wearable device). In addition, digital health interventions, such as electronic health records, decision support tools, mobile phone apps and social media are improving access to palliative care information. Children and young people with serious illness are active users of social media and can use digital technologies with ease due to their use of smart phone technologies and engagement with online gaming (Peat et al., 2019). The transference of some cares and support to digital interfaces may be more relevant and of interest to children and young people with serious illness than what support was available to them pre pandemic. There remains however, a dearth of literature around this subject with studies needed to explore to what extent digital technologies and digital health interventions can improve quality of life and support children and young people's palliative care provision (Peat et al., 2019).

Chapter summary

The anthropologic framework of liminality and the phenomenological understanding of embodiment can assist us in understanding the lived experiences of individuals with palliative care needs and their families. This understanding of individuals lived experiences can also assist health and social care professionals in their approaches to care in helping them provide an empathic presence, understanding the liminal nature of the space and time in which individuals bodily reside.

Professionals can encourage meaningful reflection, exploring issues of psychosocial and spiritual identity and can help families make sense and meaning out of their boundedness, and to experiences pertinent to total pain and quality of life. This can help individuals and families feel more sense of worth and become accepting of their condition or plight. When individuals and families accept where they are at, it is at that place they can begin to accept the end point of the journey and be more focused on the life to live over the life to lose.

Serious illness for all involved is traumatic, instrumental support for individuals and family carers can help buffer the stress of what is an emotionally intense period of their lives. With daily exposure to death and dying, professionals also need sources of support to enhance their resilience. Being able to see a silver living through meaning making can influence post traumatic growth and support acute and longer-term wellbeing for individuals facing shortened lives, families and health and social care professionals. In times of humanitarian crises such as the COVID-19 pandemic and war, the coming together of families and communities to care, can support a shared wellbeing and a resiliency outcome.

This is not withstanding the emotional scarring that can and does occur, but a common purpose and experience can lead to a network of support that helps us to transcend to better times ahead.

Key issues

1. At first the palliative care world can feel alien for individuals and families.
2. Although the experience of serious illness has many challenging junctures, the interdisciplinary palliative care team, families and communities can come together to provide support to ease the suffering or help with the adjustment to new ways of being.
3. The experience of serious illness and supporting someone with palliative care needs is subjective and embodied.
4. Pain within the context of serious illness is referred to as total pain – the embodied and multifaceted nature of the pain experience for individuals is captured by this terminology.
5. Pain assessment and management becomes mainstream to the palliative care experience. Different techniques and tools are available for different populations. Quality of life and health related quality of life are related considerations. It is recognised that fear and uncertainty can impact on these global outcomes. Furthermore, perceived hopelessness and a perceived loss of self can lead to mental health difficulties and for some a desire for a hastened death.
6. Dignity conserving practices that encourage individuals to live more in the moment can help those struggling to think about the future.
7. Although there are aspects of living with serious illness perceived as negative, there can be experiences that lead to psychological and spiritual growth, enabling individuals to find new meaning and value in life.
8. In times of humanitarian crises the practices of palliative care can benefit others but lead to changes in support and care for those living with serious illness. The Covid-19 pandemic led to many children and young people with serious illness shielding and feeling isolated from health and social care professional support. The increased use of digital health technologies arose and may continue to develop post pandemic.

Box 6.1 Reflective questions

1. No two individuals will experience serious illness or palliative care in the same way. Can you consider the breadth of factors that can impact on experiences for individuals with different conditions? Family dynamics? Developmental stages? With different socio-economic backgrounds?

2. Can you reflect on any 'silver lining' experience that has evolved for you following a personal or familial challenge? Or that you have observed in your practice? What influenced this outcome?
3. Can you see how and in what ways digital health technologies may benefit children and young people with serious illness?

References

Adams, J.G. and Walls, R.M., 2020. Supporting the health care workforce during the COVID-19 global epidemic. *Jama*, *323*(15), pp.1439–1440.

Anand, K.S., Grunau, R.E. and Oberlander, T.F., 1997. Developmental character and long-term consequences of pain in infants and children. *Child and Adolescent Psychiatric Clinics of North America*, *6*(4), pp.703–724.

Bates, A.T. and Kearney, J.A., 2015. Understanding death with limited experience in life: dying children's and adolescents' understanding of their own terminal illness and death. *Current Opinion in Supportive and Palliative Care*, *9*(1), p.40.

Bauman, Z., 1992. *Mortality, Immortality and Other Life Strategies*. Stanford University Press.

Bergner, M., 1989. Quality of life, health status, and clinical research. *Medical Care*, *27*(3), Supplement: Advances in Health Status Assessment: Conference Proceedings, pp. S148–S156.

Bluvstein, I., Moravchick, L., Sheps, D., Schreiber, S. and Bloch, M., 2013. Posttraumatic growth, posttraumatic stress symptoms and mental health among coronary heart disease survivors. *Journal of Clinical Psychology in Medical Settings*, *20*(2), pp.164–172.

Bom, J. and Stöckel, J., 2021. Is the grass greener on the other side? The health impact of providing informal care in the UK and the Netherlands. *Social Science & Medicine*, *269*, p.113562.

Bom, J., Bakx, P., Schut, F. and Van Doorslaer, E., 2019. The impact of informal caregiving for older adults on the health of various types of caregivers: a systematic review. *The Gerontologist*, *59*(5), pp. e629–e642.

Boucher, N.A. and Johnson, K.S., 2021. Cultivating cultural competence: how are hospice staff being educated to engage racially and ethnically diverse patients?. *American Journal of Hospice and Palliative Medicine®*, *38*(2), pp.169–174.

Bury, M., 1982. Chronic illness as biographical disruption. *Sociology of Health & Illness*, *4*(2), pp.167–182.

Chambers, C.T., Reid, G.J., Craig, K.D., McGrath, P.J. and Finley, G.A., 1998. Agreement between child and parent reports of pain. *The Clinical Journal of Pain*, *14*(4), pp.336–342.

Charmaz, K., 2002. Stories and silences: Disclosures and self in chronic illness. *Qualitative Inquiry*, *8*(3), pp.302–328.

Chen, J.A., Rosenberg, L.B., Schulman, B.J., Alpert, J.E. and Waldinger, R.J., 2018. Re-examining the call of duty: teaching boundaries in medical school. *Academic Medicine*, *93*(11), pp.1624–1630.

Cherny, N.I., 2007. Palliative care in situations of conflict: lessons from Jerusalem. *American Journal of Hospice and Palliative Medicine®*, *23*(6), pp.469–474.

Chochinov, H.M., 2002. Dignity-conserving care – a new model for palliative care: helping the patient feel valued. *Jama*, *287*(17), pp.2253–2260.

Chochinov, H.M., Hack, T., Hassard, T., Kristjanson, L.J., McClement, S. and Harlos, M., 2004. Dignity and psychotherapeutic considerations in end-of-life care. *Journal of Palliative Care, 20*(3), pp.134–141.

Cohen, S.R. and Leis, A., 2002. What determines the quality of life of terminally ill cancer patients from their own perspective? *Journal of Palliative Care, 18*(1), pp.48–58.

Cohen-Gogo, S., Marioni, G., Laurent, S., Gaspar, N., Semeraro, M., Gabolde, M., Dufour, C., Valteau-Couanet, D. and Brugières, L., 2011. End of life care in adolescents and young adults with cancer: experience of the adolescent unit of the Institut Gustave Roussy. *European Journal of Cancer, 47*(18), pp.2735–2741.

Cousineau, N., McDowell, I., Hotz, S. and Hébert, P., 2003. Measuring chronic patients' feelings of being a burden to their caregivers: development and preliminary validation of a scale. *Medical Care, 41*(1), pp.110–118.

Curran, K.A., 2014. Too much information – the ethics of self-disclosure. *New England Journal of Medicine, 371*(1), pp.8–9.

Downey, L., Engelberg, R.A., Curtis, J.R., Lafferty, W.E. and Patrick, D.L., 2009. Shared priorities for the end-of-life period. *Journal of Pain and Symptom Management, 37*(2), pp.175–188.

Downing, J. and Luyirika, E., 2018. Managing total pain where there is no education on pain. In: Bhatnagar, S. (Ed.), *Cancer Pain Management in Developing Countries.* Woltes Kluwer Health.

Faircloth, C.A., Boylstein, C., Rittman, M., Young, M.E. and Gubrium, J., 2004. Sudden illness and biographical flow in narratives of stroke recovery. *Sociology of Health & Illness, 26*(2), pp.242–261.

Fann, J.R., Ell, K. and Sharpe, M., 2012. Integrating psychosocial care into cancer services. *Journal of Clinical Oncology, 30*(11), pp.1178–1186.

Fletcher, P.C., 2011. My child has cancer: finding the silver lining in every mother's nightmare. *Issues in Comprehensive Pediatric Nursing, 34*(1), pp.40–55.

Geng, H.M., Chuang, D.M., Yang, F., Yang, Y., Liu, W.M., Liu, L.H. and Tian, H.M., 2018. Prevalence and determinants of depression in caregivers of cancer patients: A systematic review and meta-analysis. *Medicine, 97*(39), pp.e11863.

Giddens, A., 1991. *Modernity and Self-Identity: Self and Society in the Late Modern Age.* Stanford University Press.

Griffin, I.S. and Fentiman, M., 2002. 17. Psychosocial problems following a diagnosis of breast cancer. *International Journal of Clinical Practice, 56*(9), pp.672–675.

Heidegger, M., 1996. *Being and Time: A Translation of Sein und Zeit.* SUNY Press.

Hoffmaster, B., 2011. The rationality and morality of dying children. *Hastings center report, 41*(6), pp.30–42.

Husebo, B.S., Strand, L.I., Moe-Nilssen, R., Husebo, S.B., Snow, A.L. and Ljunggren, A.E., 2007. Mobilization-Observation-Behavior-Intensity-Dementia Pain Scale (MOBID): development and validation of a nurse-administered pain assessment tool for use in dementia. *Journal of Pain and Symptom Management, 34*(1), pp.67–80.

Husserl, E., 1983. *Ideas pertaining to a pure phenomenology and to a phenomenological philosophy: First book: General introduction to a pure phenomenology* (Vol. 2). Springer Science & Business Media.

Hvidt, E.A., 2017. The existential cancer journey: Travelling through the intersubjective structure of homeworld/alienworld. *Health: 21*(4), pp.375–391.

Karnofsky, D., and Burchenal, J., 1949. The clinical evaluation of chemotherapeutic agents in cancer. In: C. M. Macleod (Ed.), *Evaluation of chemotherapeutic agents.* (pp. 191–205). Columbia University Press.

Keenan, P. and Mac Dermott, C., 2016. How nurses grieve for children who die in their care. *Learning Disability Practice*, *19*(3), pp.16–22.

Kleinman, A., 1997. 'Everything that really matters': social suffering, subjectivity, and the remaking of human experience in a disordering world. *Harvard Theological Review*, *90*(3), pp.315–336.

Kluetz, P.G., Slagle, A., Papadopoulos, E.J., Johnson, L.L., Donoghue, M., Kwitkowski, V.E., Chen, W.H., Sridhara, R., Farrell, A.T., Keegan, P. and Kim, G., 2016. Focusing on core patient-reported outcomes in cancer clinical trials: symptomatic adverse events, physical function, and disease-related symptoms. *Clinical Cancer Research*, *22*(7), pp.1553–1558.

Lussier, M.T. and Richard, C., 2007. Self-disclosure during medical encounters. *Canadian Family Physician*, *53*(3), pp.421–422.

Maben, J. and Bridges, J., 2020. Covid-19: Supporting nurses' psychological and mental health. *Journal of Clinical Nursing*, pp. Accepted-Article.

Marmot, M., 2020. Health equity in England: The Marmot review 10 years on. *BMJ*, *368*: m693.

McDaniel, S.H., Beckman, H.B., Morse, D.S., Silberman, J., Seaburn, D.B. and Epstein, R.M., 2007. Physician self-disclosure in primary care visits: enough about you, what about me? *Archives of Internal Medicine*, *167*(12), pp.1321–1326.

Melzack, R. and Wall, P.D., 1965. Pain mechanisms: a new theory: a gate control system modulates sensory input from the skin before it evokes pain perception and response. *Science*, *150*(3699), pp.971–979.

Melzack, R., 1982. Recent concepts of pain. *Journal of Medicine*, *13*(3), pp.147–160.

Mercadante, S., Adile, C., Ferrera, P., Giuliana, F., Terruso, L. and Piccione, T., 2020. Palliative care in the time of COVID-19. *Journal of Pain and Symptom Management*, *60*(2), pp. e79–e80.

Mercadante, S., Giuliana, F., Terruso, L. and Albegiani, G., 2020. Hospice care pathways and COVID-19. *BMJ Supportive & Palliative Care*, Published Online First: 17 September 2020. doi: 10.1136/bmjspcare-2020-002505.

Merleau-Ponty, M. and Smith, C., 1962. *Phenomenology of Perception* (Vol. 26). London: Routledge.

Merleau-Ponty, M., 1968. *The Visible and the Invisible: Followed by Working Notes*. Northwestern University Press.

Muni, S., Engelberg, R.A., Treece, P.D., Dotolo, D. and Curtis, J.R., 2011. The influence of race/ethnicity and socioeconomic status on end-of-life care in the ICU. *Chest*, *139*(5), pp.1025–1033.

Nicholas Dionne-Odom, J., Hooker, S.A., Bekelman, D., Ejem, D., McGhan, G., Kitko, L., Strömberg, A., Wells, R., Astin, M., Metin, Z.G. and Mancarella, G., 2017. Family caregiving for persons with heart failure at the intersection of heart failure and palliative care: a state-of-the-science review. *Heart Failure Reviews*, *22*(5), pp.543–557.

Nilmanat, K., Chailungka, P., Phungrassami, T., Promnoi, C., Tulathamkit, K., Noo-urai, P. and Phattaranavig, S., 2010. Living with suffering as voiced by Thai patients with terminal advanced cancer. *International Journal of Palliative Nursing*, *16*(8), pp.393–399.

Nishio, M., Kimura, H., Ogomori, K. and Ogata, K., 2017. Emotional and instrumental support influencing male caregivers for people with dementia living at home. *Journal of Rural Medicine*, *12*(1), pp.20–27.

Nouvet, E, Sivaram, M, Bezanson, K, et al. 2018. Palliative care in humanitarian crises: a review of the literature. *J Int Humanit Action*, 3(1), p.5.

Office for National Statistics, 2020, Deaths in care homes www.ons.gov.uk/aboutus/transparencyandgovernance/freedomofinformationfoi/covid19deathsincarehomes (accessed 3 June 2022)
Office for National Statistics, 2021, Deaths in care homes www.ons.gov.uk/aboutus/transparencyandgovernance/freedomofinformationfoi/covid19deathsincarehomes2021 (accessed 3 June 2022)
Parpa, E., Tsilika, E., Galanos, A., Nikoloudi, M. and Mystakidou, K., 2019. Depression as mediator and or moderator on the relationship between hopelessness and patients' desire for hastened death. *Supportive Care in Cancer*, *27*(11), pp.4353–4358.
Peat, G., Rodriguez, A. and Smith, J., 2019. Social media use in adolescents and young adults with serious illnesses: an integrative review. *BMJ Supportive & Palliative Care*, *9*(3), pp.235–244.
Periyakoil, V.S., Chmura Kraemer, H. and Noda, A., 2009. Creation and the empirical validation of the dignity card-sort tool to assess factors influencing erosion of dignity at life's end. *Journal of Palliative Medicine*, *12*(12), pp.1125–1130.
Reid, F., 2013. Grief and the experiences of nurses providing palliative care to children and young people at home. *Nursing Children and Young People*, *25*(9), pp.31–36.
Rietjens, J., Korfage, I. and Taubert, M., 2021. Advance care planning: the future. *BMJ Supportive & Palliative Care*, *11*(1), pp.89–91.
Roberts, J., Fenton, G. and Barnard, M., 2015. Developing effective therapeutic relationships with children, young people and their families. *Nursing Children and Young People*, *27*(4).
Rodriguez, A. 2009. 'We are here for a good time not a long time': Being and acring for a child with a life limiting condition. Doctoral Thesis. University of Huddersfield http://eprints.hud.ac.uk/id/eprint/6963/
Rodriguez, A. and King, N., 2009. The lived experience of parenting a child with a life-limiting condition: a focus on the mental health realm. *Palliative & Supportive Care*, 7(1), pp.7–12.
Rodriguez, A. and King, N., 2014. Sharing the care: the key-working experiences of professionals and the parents of life-limited children. *International Journal of Palliative Nursing*, *20*(4), pp.165–171.
Royal College of Nursing, 2021. New nursing education module www.rcn.org.uk/news-and-events/news/uk-rcn-launches-online-learning-tool-supporting-nursing-staff-new-to-critical-care-080121 (accessed 3 June, 2022).
Sabat, S.R. and Collins, M., 1999. Intact social, cognitive ability, and selfhood: A case study of Alzheimer's disease. *American Journal of Alzheimer's Disease*, *14*(1), pp.11–19.
Schag, C. Coscarelli, Richard L. Heinrich, and Patricia A. Ganz. 1984. Karnofsky performance status revisited: reliability, validity, and guidelines. *Journal of Clinical Oncology*, *2*(3), pp. 187–193.
Sese D, Makhoul, A., Hoeksema, L. and Shoemaker, L., 2020. The role of palliative care in COVID-19. *Cleve Clin J Med*, doi: 10.3949/ccjm.87a.ccc036. Epub ahead of print. PMID: 32471812.
Smith, J. and Aloudat, T., 2017. Palliative care in humanitarian medicine. *Palliative Medicine*, *31*(2), pp.99–101.
Steinbock, A.J., 1995. *Home and Beyond: Generative Phenomenology after Husserl*. Northwestern University Press.
Tedeschi, R.G., Shakespeare-Finch, J., Taku, K. and Calhoun, L.G., 2018. *Posttraumatic Growth: Theory, Research, and Applications*. Routledge.

The International Association for the Study of Pain (IASP), 2022., Definition of pain. www.iasp-pain.org/resources/terminology/#pain (accessed 3 June 2022).

van Laarhoven, H.W., Schilderman, J., Bleijenberg, G., Donders, R., Vissers, K.C., Verhagen, C.A. and Prins, J.B., 2011. Coping, quality of life, depression, and hopelessness in cancer patients in a curative and palliative, end-of-life care setting. *Cancer Nursing*, *34*(4), pp.302–314.

van Mol, M., Wagener, S., Rietjens, J. and den Uil, C.A., 2022. Symptoms of psychological distress among bereaved relatives of deceased patients in the intensive care unit during the first COVID-19 wave. *Intensive Care Medicine*, *48*(4), pp.491–492.

Volker, D.L. and Wu, H.L., 2011. Cancer patients' preferences for control at the end of life. *Qualitative Health Research*, *21*(12), pp.1618–1631.

Wales, J., 2019. Last song – sharing humanity while maintaining boundaries. *The New England Journal of Medicine*, *381*(20), pp.1894–1895.

Weis, J. and Boehncke, A., 2011. Psychological comorbidity in patients with cancer. *Bundesgesundheitsblatt, Gesundheitsforschung, Gesundheitsschutz*, *54*(1), pp.46–51.

Williams, S. and Bendelow, G., 1998. In search of the «missing body. *Pain, suffering and the (post) modern condition*», in Scambler Graham & Paul Higgs ed, Modernity, medicine and Health. New York: Routledge, pp.125–146.

Yancu, C.N., Farmer, D.F. and Leahman, D., 2010. Barriers to hospice use and palliative care services use by African American adults. *American Journal of Hospice and Palliative Medicine®*, *27*(4), pp.248–253.

Zanatta, F., Maffoni, M. and Giardini, A., 2020. Resilience in palliative healthcare professionals: a systematic review. *Supportive Care in Cancer*, *28*(3), pp.971–978.

7 Dying well

Children and young people's end of life care

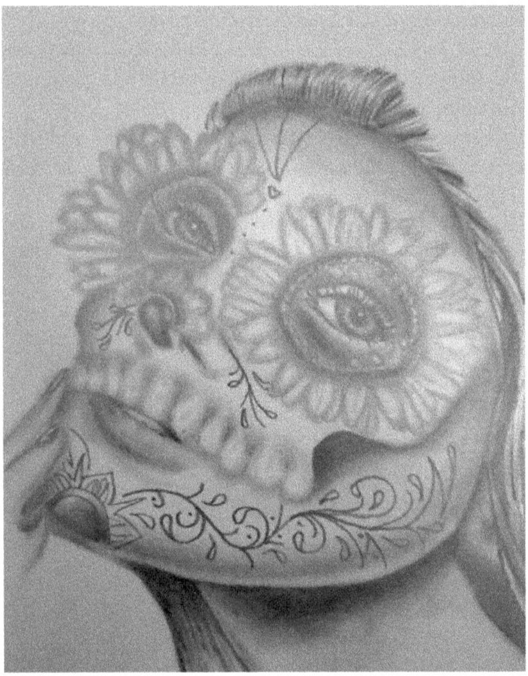

Figure 7.1 Photograph of artwork by Iris Rodriguez. Photograph taken by Alison Rodriguez.

Introduction

The concept of 'a good death' was first addressed by Weisman in 1972 with his work on the 'appropriate death', that he defined as a process whereby all involved know that death is imminent, and that the dying person has resolved

DOI: 10.4324/9781003340287-8

any socioemotional or practical concerns. Over time scholars began referring to the 'good death' with the same sentiment. The conception of a good death is now somewhat dated as we understand that the perception of someone dying well is both complex and relative to the unique preferences of the individual who is dying.

As individuals live with serious illness, palliative care in all its guises, recognises that if we do have the gift of time, then the physical and emotional comfort we can gain from our surroundings, both environmentally and in terms of supportive family/friends and professionals, is of paramount importance to us and can contribute to living with a more positive mindset up until death.

> Simone de Beauvoir wrote that *'There is no such thing as a natural death … for every man his death is an accident, and, even if he knows it and consents to it, it remains an unjustifiable violation'.*
>
> (1966, p106)

Individuals do not relent immediately to the prospect of dying; it takes time to develop a level of acceptance that one's life is soon to end. Some individuals really struggle to get to a point of acceptance, simply because they are frightened. They fear the dying process and of what physical changes may happen. Being given a shortened life prognosis effects the individual's sense of their secure being in the world, more so if they feel they have not yet had the opportunity to fully live out their lives, maybe because of their age/developmental stage or life opportunities.

We all have hopes and dreams that we live towards, and these are disrupted or abolished following the knowledge of impending death. Personal and social identities are scripted around who we are in the world, however with the onset of serious illness, advancing disease or increasing disability, we begin to reconfigure our 'selves' and promote the aspects of our being that we want to be recognised by or known for. Once we are dying, we become a 'dying person' and in trying to identify with that status, we are left to relate to the scripts or narratives of that status as relevant to the culture we belong to. These same scripts also help us to negotiate how to die well (Seale, 1998).

The open communication or model of truth telling advocated in many resource rich countries and palliative care, whereby the individual with serious illness is provided with as much information as possible about their condition and its trajectory, is a modern directive. Up until 1970 it was routine practice for professionals to not disclose to individuals their life shortening prognosis. Weisman (1972) lifted the veil on this practice and argued that when professionals are not honest with individuals, saying nothing about impending death, then they increase individual existential distress because individuals are often silently aware that they are not going to recover. If a life shortening prognosis is confirmed it can then be a source of mental ease, not just for individuals but also for their families, who can then be open with the individual in supporting and meeting their needs.

At the same time of the move in attitudes towards being more open with individuals about their dying, it was realised in health care that dying people also needed professional expertise in care and support, not least to support the dying process.

The achievement of a 'good death' was central to the philosophy of the hospice movement and palliative care, which stipulates that a good death includes:

- The aggressive treatment of signs and symptoms of discomfort
- Exploring the impact of illness on quality of life and improve coping
- Being present through the individual and family experience at the end of life, and
- Supporting individuals to not have to live with the fear of loss of dignity, dying alone, or being in pain (Gazelle, 2003).

There is also a wealth of lay literature that illustrates contemporary attitudes towards 'dying well.' For example, in 'The Last Lecture' (Zaslow and Pausch, 2014), Randy Pausch, who was a prominent engineering lecturer in USA, embraces the media and talks about his diagnosis of pancreatic cancer and life shortening prognosis. His target message was to embrace the life you have, every moment of that life because *'time is all you have…and you may find one day that you have less than you think.'*

Steve Jobs, an iconic businessperson and founder of apple computers Inc., similarly at Stanford University and following his cancer diagnosis, stated that death is '*very likely the single best invention of life'* and talked about how post diagnosis his focus was on the most meaningful aspects of life for him.

These mediatised examples of individuals living towards their deaths, highlight contemporary constructs of personal experience and how in many resource rich countries, we value the courage of individuals positivity towards their death (Meier et al., 2016).

The thought of a 'good' death for many however, remains incomprehensible.

How can anyone's experience toward death be positive or good?

Perhaps this use of terminology is both outdated and inappropriate?

However, just as we hope that our entry into this world is fluid, natural and painless, many of us desire that our death and dying will have similar qualities.

At the end of life, we may want to be supported by the ones we love, alongside those placed in a professional capacity to care. This could be one characteristic of what we perceive of as a 'good' death. However, if we ponder further and consider our expectations of a 'good' death, we may begin to consider a list of factors characteristic of good end of life care. In the immediacy of our thoughts, a hastened death could be desired, but as we think more deeply about the matter, a better death might be one whereby we know it is coming, and one where we have the gift of time to say goodbye.

Death and dying is synonymous with thoughts of physical pain.

Would we want to be free of physical pain?

Would this then be replaced with existential pain?

There is anxiety about not knowing what to expect.

Experiencing the fear of death and dying can also involve the emotional torment of leaving loved ones behind. Therefore, the 'good' death is emotionally all encompassing.

In exploring the literature around this subject area and considering both the cultural and spiritual needs of different age and disease groups, it is useful to reflect on how individuals might want their deaths to be and how they want their palliative and end of life care to be, if gifted with time. Decision making may alter with the stage of the illness trajectory or indeed level of capacity. Individual biographies, social and personal identities may each also impact on wishes. As such, it can be appreciated that a multitude of needs, hopes and desires are likely to be mused over by those facing the end of their lives and their families (Steinhauser et al., 2000; Beckstrand et al., 2006; Weiner et al, 2022).

In children and young people's palliative care much support is offered to individuals who have conditions from birth but may be expected to live for many years with serious illness. Their timelines may be difficult to determine, and they may live through many peaks and troughs with respect to wellness, sometimes being close to death at several junctures. And yet still death may come as a surprise and especially for the family when it does happen.

In children and young people's palliative care the over riding focus is on quality of life and on living in the moment. The thinking about dying is not something to muse over for families and professionals alike, it is too difficult. Until perhaps there is a realisation of increased frailty, the person has encountered a sudden decline in health or on review, or the person appears to be living beyond their years of expectation, why spend too much time on thinking about the end of life?

Many issues are implicated in this approach and that we have covered elsewhere in the book, with respect to truth telling and the therapeutic benefit of meaning making, and legacy leaving and also impacts of living with serious illness and a life shortening prognosis on the mental health and wellbeing of the child, young person and family. It is possible that to achieve the 'living well' can incorporate thinking about the 'dying well' too. To achieve this, structured interventions could assist the challenging conversations to occur, for children and young people to not need to think about opportune moments to ask a carer about if they are dying and what might that involve. If communication is afforded to children and young people in age-appropriate ways, allowing them to talk about end of life wishes and concerns then it is possible that later emotional suffering can be lessened. There remains however much more research needed in this area of challenge for children, young people and families in palliative care.

Cultural conceptions of death

There are two universal facts to our human existence, one we are all born and two we all die. We welcome each new life into our worlds with much joy and excitement and often lots of planning and preparing. Death on the other hand is something we do not ruminate on, talk very little about and spend little effort planning for, especially if we or someone close to us is not living through a life threatening or life limiting illness. Even if a person does have such a condition, this provides no guarantee that death is something they want to plan or look forward to. As such, death denial can be amassed amongst varied communities. In addition, what we constitute as death can also be multifaceted and is debated by different scholars and cultural perspectives. Differences in definition can also affect how we may perceive death and dying.

The difficulty we have in understanding how death and dying can be viewed so differently amongst people, is further complicated by the fact that there is no universal consensus on how we should define bodily death. For over a century the clinical definition of death centred on there being an absence of a heart beating and a respiratory system functioning. However, as we have made medical advances our vital signs can now be managed by technology. As a result, a modified definition of death has been developed to include whole brain death. Coupled with this modern understanding of death is a list of criteria that must be met so a person can be determined deceased:

1. *Absence of spontaneous response to any stimuli.*
2. *Completely unresponsive to even the most painful stimuli.*
3. *Lack of spontaneous respiration for at least one hour.*
4. *Absence of postural activity, swallowing, yawning, or vocalising.*
5. *No eye movements, blinking, or pupil responses.*
6. *A flat electroencephalogram (EEG) for at least 10 minutes.*
7. *A total absence of motor reflexes.*
8. *No change in the above criteria if tested again after 24 hours.* (Gardiner et al., 2012; Association of Ambulance Chief Executives and Joint Royal Colleges Ambulances Liaison Committee (JRCALC), 2019; President's Commission for the Study of Ethical Problems in Medicine and Biomedical and Behavioural Research, 1981, p. 4).

This definition is representative of western thought and follows on from biomedical presumptions. However, across cultures there remains no global agreement on such a biomedical definition. Some add that the no brain activity needs to also state that there must be no activity in the brain cortex and brain stem. Our brain cortexes provide us with executive functioning, we can identify as conscious human beings because of the functions allowed by the cortex. Alternatively, the brain stem controls vegetative function such as breathing. When our cortex's fail, we become unconscious but if our brainstems remain active then we can still breathe, and our hearts will still beat. However, if our cortex's have 'died' then we will remain in a persistent vegetative state and will not redeem our consciousness. Such a state can be induced because of a major head injury, a stoppage in blood flow to the brain or even intoxication from drugs overdoses. Although the persistent vegetative condition is irreversible, those affected are not presumed dead if we use the current biomedical and mainstream definition of death. In a persistent and vegetative state, the individual is technologically alive, and in a state of being alive but without awareness, a state of increasing prevalence due to our increasing use of modern-day technologies.

This situation can be extremely stressful and emotionally upsetting for families, not least because it poses so many ethical challenges. As a result, there has been a call from both scientific and philosophical expertise to use the death of the cortical brain as the standard for death and not the whole brain definition. With the argument being that without the capacity for consciousness then we are dead (Truog, 2004). As such, an individual assessed to be in a permanent coma and who is considered to now be in a persistent vegetative state would be declared dead. The same person would not be declared dead using the whole brain standard. This is just our western biomedical understanding; things can get even more complicated when we consider non-western and religious conceptualisations.

For example, people from some areas of the South Pacific believe that when a person is ill or asleep, the life of them drains away, and so they can 'die' many times before their ultimate physical or bodily death. Therefore, in these communities, a person would be presumed dead without needing to apply the whole brain or cortical brain death standard. Differences in cultural understandings continue when the person is dead (as per the western definitions) irrespective of the detail of how that death is defined. For example, Hindus like Buddhists envision a circular pattern of life and death (samsara). The four noble truths of Buddhist teachings also infer the contemplation of suffering (*sutras*). The *Upajjhatthana Sutra*, often referred to as the 'Five Remembrances' is believed to typify our human mortality:

1. I will age
2. I will become ill
3. I will die
4. I will become separated from significant others
5. I am responsible for my actions (Langer, 2007).

It is routine for Buddhists to contemplate death. Their belief system advocates that there is an afterlife that we will visit many times and where we will manifest into different forms. The goal for Buddhists is nirvana, to be lifted from the prevailing cycle of birth, suffering, death, and rebirth (Gyatso, 1995, Langer, 2007).

Different pre death rituals exist across Buddhist communities however the person's bodily condition prior to their death is of importance to all. For example, if the dying person has elevated levels of death anxiety, then it is believed that their rebirth could also be traumatic (Kramer, 1988). The dying should also refrain from treatments that could alter their consciousness or mental clarity because much weight is held on the dying to have the ability to maintain their virtuous thinking because such will influence their transition into death and again their rebirth (Gyatso and Jinpa, 1995). The 'good' death is one that takes place in the home, surrounded by family, friends and monks reciting the sutras to promote peace at death and transition. Following death great cares are given to the body. The body is washed by male family members, wrapped and thumbs and toes are bound with the hair of another family member. A coin is put inside the deceased's mouth and on their head, with flowers placed at their side (Kramer, 1988). The body does not leave the family for four days and on that day the body is cremated. In this time friends also visit. At the cremation and for several days following, monks pray to influence a good life transition (Kramer, 1988).

This is opposite to the Christian view, where death happens to us just once.

The New Testament of the bible details the teachings of Jesus Christ. It is believed we all die because of the original sin, but our death is a temporary separation of spirit and body. In the second coming of Christ, we will be resurrected. The nature of our dying can also be considered resultant of our life sins; therefore, health and social care professionals need to be ready to support some Christians who may perceive their illness as punishment and may be suffering elevated levels of guilt and fear for what may become of them following their death (Braun and Zir, 2001). A 'good' Christian death involves being spiritually prepared, having resolve in interpersonal relationships (forgiveness) and reconciling sins, such may promote the transition to heaven and not an encounter with purgatory or an eternity in hell (Braun and Zir, 2001).

The teachings of Islam are revealed by God through the prophet Muhammed. However, there are slight differences in the ways different Muslim communities interpret the Islamic teachings. The term 'vernacular Islam' has been used to describe the varied interpretations (Flueckiger, 2006). In the medical literature, Muslim professionals support the pharmacological treatment of pain (Gatrad, 1994). However, Islamic law (Sharia) does not permit the use of narcotics to hasten death and euthanasia is not supported. The management of pain and other symptoms must not interfere with the individual's ability to pray and engage in Islamic ritual, even at the very end of their lives. It is believed that these prayers and rituals are needed to support the soul's journey into the afterlife and later resurrection (Abu-Ras and Laird, 2011). The good death for Muslims is very much a social happening. Family members are expected to perform cares to the individual. In times of consciousness, family and friends will support the individual to pray and to also reflect upon their lives lived. Once the individual is unconscious, together family and friends hold prayers and call for forgiveness and protection of the individual's soul. This care continues with the preparation of the body for burial. Families wash and cloth the deceased and participate in spiritual contemplation. This is because the Islamic belief is that the person's soul does not leave its body until the time of burial (Gatrad and Sheikh, 2002).

When death is imminent, individuals who belong to the Jewish faith also recite specific prayers and families accompany the dying individual as they die. This is deemed an act of respect. Following the death, certain procedures must be carried out also by the family. The eyes and mouth are shut, and a sheet is positioned to cover the face. The body must be positioned on their back and looking towards the door. Burning candles are positioned at the head of the body. In addition, any poured water in the home, for example, in glasses, jugs or vases need to be poured away and any mirrors in the home covered. The Rabbi is then summonsed to visit the deceased and inform the Chevra Kaddish (Holy Society). The Chevra Kaddish is a group of individuals within the community who are tasked with the duty of body preparation. This involves reciting certain prayers, cleaning, and dressing the body. From the point of death until burial, the deceased must not be left alone. A shomer (watcher) is called upon to be always at the side of the body (Bauer-Wu, et al., 2007).

Jewish funerals like Islamic ones are to be conducted as quickly as possible, ideally within 24 hours of death. The funeral involves prayers in the funeral home or at the graveyard. The rituals that may be observed in other funeral types are disallowed in Jewish funerals, for example open coffins, flowers, music, and cremation.

Irrespective of how death is defined, each culture has notions of how death ought to occur and coupled with that, how cares of the deceased need to be conducted. Notably, the 'good' dying or end of life care transcends to the 'good' death which transcends to the 'good' care of the deceased. The processes involved are both personal and social.

Kellehear (1990) delineates the 'acceptable death' from the 'good death' for the person who is dying. An 'acceptable' death is considered peaceful, routinised and with little emotionality. Such a death resembles those that can be observed in the hospital wards of resource rich countries. In contrast, the 'good' death allows room for social adjustments and accommodates the end of life wishes of the dying individual and their family. This might mean accommodating the individuals need to say goodbye to certain people and to complete other tasks that will help family and friends cope with their death. Completing certain tasks and finishing life business is important in some communities. A good death is construed when the deceased is perceived to have completed their life tasks and resolved any conflicts with others. However, in other communities a 'good' death is one that can only be achieved by the completion of a period of service to one's country or religion – they must be a martyr (Rosenblatt, 2008).

Such different conceptualisations of what constitutes a 'good' death also affects how individuals conduct themselves through life and how they perceive or anticipate their dying. Religious affiliation provides social support, but religious guidance can help individuals make sense of life, death, and life after death. Despite the noted nuances, all the major religions desire a peaceful death and discourage any attempt to hasten death. Indeed, the sacred writings of Judaism, Buddhism, Hinduism, Islam, and Christianity each reject euthanasia but allow the relief of suffering at the end-of-life.

Death anxiety: the fear of death

Irrespective of cultural heritage and religious belief systems, the most common response to the thought of one's own death, or the death of other loved ones, is fear. Drawing on the social psychological perspective, researchers have referred to terror management theory to enhance our understanding of death anxiety (Burke et al., 2010; Tam, 2013). Terror management theory (Pyszczynski, et al., 2015) details that animals have an evolutionary and instinctual drive for self-preservation. Humans also possess this drive and coupled with their advanced cognitive abilities, they can develop a self-awareness and ability to consider and prepare for their futures. These instinctual qualities enable us to envisage death and to accept that such could happen to us at any given time.

However, as human beings we possess a conflict between self-preservation and death awareness and the perceived inevitability and unpredictability can induce both anxiety and terror. The terror management perspective argues that much of our human behaviour that is to our avail is to negotiate these givens and to deal with the anxiety and terror of them. Although, those who are very anxious about death will grapple to engage in any death preventing measures available and will try to stay alive at all costs. This endless grappling for cure or recovery can lead to further physical and mental issues.

Aside from how we may deal with death anxiety, we need to be mindful that the concept of death anxiety itself is complex and difficult to define. It can incorporate fear of one's own death, the death of others and fear of the dying process. Each element of fear can be further analysed at different personal and social levels. What we experience and exude socially may be quite different to what we internally process and how we cope privately. Indeed, we may not be conscious of how our death anxieties are acted out.

Death anxiety is often manifested through death avoidance (Kastenbaum, 2000). Some people are so uncomfortable with death, they will avoid funerals and visiting the dying. This may be excused formally by work schedules and sometimes will not be a conscious action. Others can display their anxiety with constant death talk or availing themselves to risky behaviours, such as outdoor pursuits. Death anxiety can also be an explanation factor for individuals who seek out cosmetic surgery to look younger. If they look young then these individuals are more at ease with telling themselves that death could be further away from their door (Tam, 2013).

Death anxiety is evident in all communities. However, diverse cultures express various levels of intensity publicly. Societies that appear more accepting of death are labelled death affirming societies. Other cultures can be so averted to death that they are labelled as death denying cultures. The societies more accepting of death incorporate those with more Eastern or collectivist cultural beliefs. Eastern conceptions of death are to view death as a mere transition, just another fact of life (Schumaker et al., 1988). It is, however, understandable that because death anxiety is multifaceted that differences can exist across cultural and ethnic groups.

The Multidimensional Fear of Death Scale (MFODS; Hoelter, 1979; Neimeyer and Moore, 1994) was used in a study by DePaola et al. (2003). Conducted in America, the study found that there were significant differences between elderly African Americans and Caucasian Americans on various aspects of death anxiety. Caucasians scored higher on the death anxiety of the dying process scale. This could be because Caucasians are more likely to die in health organised settings. This then would mean a death not in the company of family. The result could also be explained by the fact that many older adults report feeling in pain which is not helped by medicines. And so, fear of death process can be rationalised based on already lived experiences. The African American participants showed higher levels of anxiety on the fear of the unknown, fear of consciousness when dead and fear of the body after death scales. This could be why African Americans are frequently reported to want to extend their lives using aggressive treatments, even in times of little hope. Still, they also reported very low levels of anxiety about anxiety on comfort care at the end of life. This could reside with the fact they know their families will provide them with cares and support at the end of their lives. These experiences and perceptions conveyed by older adult communities transcend to younger generations.

What factors within cultures give rise to differences in death anxiety?

Terror management theory (Pyszczynski, et al., 2015) suggests many of us have a profound fear of death. To manage this fear, individuals manage to negotiate themselves through several life worlds. They could for example have a need to believe in an afterlife to cope with the thought of human none existence. Religiosity is therefore prominent in this understanding and has been researched intensely. Indeed, those who are affiliated with religions that promote a belief in the afterlife have lower levels of global death anxiety than others. However, the role of religious affiliation in death anxiety is not yet conclusive because studies have achieved quite different findings. Duff and Hong (1995) recruited 674 older adults to a survey about death anxiety. They found that higher levels of anxiety were associated with a higher frequency of religious service attendances. The increased attendance could have been because of the death anxieties themselves but this was not determined.

In a cross-cultural and cross-religious survey of beliefs of the afterlife and death anxiety, Parsuram and Sharma (1992) discovered that Hindus (who had the highest belief in life after death) had the lowest levels of death anxiety, with Christians exhibiting the highest levels. The diversity of findings could be because most standardised measures do not allow a depth of response and few researchers include open ended questions in their surveys. Contemporary studies on death anxiety therefore need to be more ambitious to explore the underlying factors responsible for resultant scores.

An et al. (2018) completed a survey with 307 individuals with advanced cancer to explore their death anxiety. They completed standardised measures including the Death and Dying Distress Scale, the Demoralisation Scale, the modified Experiences in Close Relationships Scale, the Life Completion subscale of the Quality-of-Life Evaluation – Cancer scale, the Memorial Symptom Assessment Scale, and the Karnofsky Performance Status. They then used a structural equation model of protective and risk factors for demoralisation and death anxiety. The final model had good fit with death anxiety positively associated with demoralisation, and demoralisation positively associated with symptom burden and negatively associated with social relatedness. The findings therefore highlighted that demoralisation and death anxiety are intricately linked in individuals with advanced cancer. In those with serious illness, demoralisation is determined by feelings of hopelessness, a sense of a loss of meaning, and the sense of failure (Kissane, 2014).

Kawano (2011) used ethnographic methods to explore death anxiety and attitudes toward personal death among members of the Grave-Free Promotion Society (GFPS) in Japan. Historically the Japanese have had posthumous demands placed upon them to maintain the grave sites of their significant others. As work options have diversified and global travel has influenced overseas opportunities, maintaining traditional rituals has become increasingly difficult. Therefore, the death anxiety unveiled in this study was not relative to fear of death or dying, but of maintaining respectful rituals. This study shows that there can be quite unexpected and diverse reasons for why individuals may score high on death anxiety related measures and there is a call for research to use qualitative methods to explore in-depth the reasons for and meanings behind perceptions of death anxiety.

Palliative autonomy

Everyone, irrespective of religious affiliation or spiritual belief system desire a peaceful death, void of anxieties. Palliative care professionals are tasked with ensuring this happens and in finding diverse ways and using different means to make this happen. How health and social care professionals' action a 'good death' or 'dying well' in practice can be unique to each individual and family in their care. Traditional religions are becoming sparser and so historical rituals and responses to death and dying are not so widespread. Palliative care professionals are often called to step in and provide crucial supportive roles to human comfort and grief processes. The growing individualisation of faith, whereby individuals are increasingly selective and eclectic with their practices, means increasingly that the individuals meaning making must take prominence in cares. Professionals left to presume need on the simple basis of the individual's religious affiliation could wrongly interpret their wishes.

For some years, social scientists have explored to what extent policy makers have tried to embrace cultural diversity and capitalise on the concept of a ''good death' or 'dying well' in their end-of-life care policies and palliative care practice guidance. McNamara (2004) explored how the philosophy of a 'good death' is also tenuous with the climate of individual autonomy and choice. For example, individuals who 'choose' not to accept or refuse to talk openly about death, may be perceived to encounter a bad death from the perspective of professionals – even if the death they achieve meets their own personal needs or wishes. We assume that all adult members of contemporary western cultures desire openness and a discussion of wishes, but this does not respect the uniqueness of experience and how the philosophy of palliative care is to meet the individual needs of each individual. This example, however, identifies how the concept of a 'good death' is not just one that is owned by the individual but one that holds shared meaning and understanding for carers. Health and social care professionals and families also have a need to situate the death in their own frameworks of meaning and purpose.

For those individuals who are perceived to have endured a 'bad death' because it was sudden, drawn out or traumatic, or because their behaviour was not compliant with the good death model – embracing all that life has to offer until their demise, can induce a sense of personal failure for health and social care professionals and families and can sometimes create a crisis of talks around if there was a degree of negligence. Whereas when a death has followed good death practice expectations there appears to be a consensus that it was a job well achieved (McNamara et al. 1995). This discourse of the 'good' or 'bad' death and the attitudes and behaviours that accompany it, holds not just individuals accountable for their death and dying but health and social care professionals, carers, family, friends, neighbours, and wider society – as far as society is perceived to allow or prevent a 'good' death. Significant others engage in biographical meaning making (Brennan and Letherby, 2017), categorising aspects of death and dying as good or bad and these categories are often superfluous with how the deceased was being perceived to live out their life. If someone is extrovert in life and has many friends for example, it would seem only right that they end their lives in the company of their friends and family.

So, we can see furthermore that dying holds those close to us responsible, feeling obliged that they support us in our death desires and if those are not overtly expressed then we are left to assume that they relate to how we have lived. Dying well is aspirational and conceptions of a good death can be idealistic. A 'good death' or 'dying well' also necessitates a lot of support, and it is expected that the palliative care professional will assist individuals to accept death, that they will relieve pain and help with the biographical labour undertaken by family and friends, to help them situate the individual's death in their own life stories. As McNamara (2004, p936) notes, *'dying people are expected to live well until they die and make their own choices in this process'*.

Allan Kellehear's large study on the good death (1990) explored the predeath experiences of one hundred adults with cancer. Awareness of dying, social adjustments and personal preparations, arrangements relating to work and farewells were illustrated to be the five key features of the good death for the participants. The comprehensive study explored individual perspectives but also looked at each participant's social worlds. Kellehear derived a good death model that identified a shared understanding of death that involves public ritual which continues to prevail in many societies of today. Field (1996) accepted the robustness of the model for those with cancer disease trajectories however argued that the same may not be relevant to individuals dying from other conditions. Still, it is apparent that regardless of condition, it is awareness of one's life shortening prognosis that impacts on our being towards death. Both authors cite the seminal work of Glaser and Strauss (2017) further highlighting that if we have capacity, our scripts for dying resonate with how death is portrayed in the society or the cultures we belong. Dying well is something that assists us personally with a sense of well-being but to aide that there is a need for there also to be a social recognition of the plight. In Kearle's (1996) framework, deaths are good when *'they enhance the social solidarities or in ways contribute to the well-being of the living'* (1996, p346).

Individual autonomy and dignity

Palliative care plays an instrumental role in supporting individual's existential needs, this includes supporting the end of life wishes of individuals. Advanced care planning decisions are best conducted with time on the individual's side and preferably by a health care professional who they have built a good care relationship with (Rodriguez and King, 2014). This is done to prevent any familial and individual distress at the end of life, to support the individual's autonomy and to make them aware of the emotional and spiritual support that they will be able to access as their death becomes more imminent.

In practice, the Quality of Dying and Death questionnaire (QODD) (Downey et al., 2010) is often used to evaluate quality of death and as such could be considered a relic of the 'good death' construct. The tool contains thirty-one items, in six domains:

1. Time with the family,
2. Whole person concern,
3. Treatment preferences,
4. Autonomy,
5. Personal relationships, and
6. Personal concerns.

These domains relate more to the psychological, social, and spiritual, than the more physical symptoms and demands of dying.

In support of the historical studies already outlined, several more recent studies have listed what health and social care professionals perceive as 'good dying' and they are incumbent with what it also commonly perceived as good end of life care (Truog et al., 2008). The Hartford foundation recently conducted a quantitative survey identifying that physicians were motivated to discuss openly with individuals their end-of-life care for a number of key reasons:

1. To meet the values and wishes of individuals and families
2. To limit unwanted treatments
3. To heighten care satisfaction
4. To save cost
5. To increasing the use of hospice care.

One distinct finding however was that most respondents confessed that they had not discussed with individuals, issues around their end-of-life care (Hartford Foundation, 2016). Other studies have also noted this practice, physicians especially delay conversations of this nature because they worry that such will impact upon hope and such will have detriment to the individual's holistic wellbeing (Mack et al., 2012).

As compared with professionals, it is argued that families desire a more comprehensive approach to end-of-life care. A study by Singer et al. (1999) shifted the goal posts for research in this area and researched perceptions of quality end of life care from the individual's perspectives. They identified five key factors:

1. To achieve adequate pain and symptom management.
2. To avoid an unneeded extending of the dying process.
3. To achieving a sense of control.
4. To relieve burden.
5. To strengthen existent relationships with loved ones.

Following on from this work, Teno et al. (2004) summarised individual's expectations of health and social care professionals to promote high-quality end-of-life care:

1. To provide physical and emotional support.
2. To encourage shared decision-making.
3. To give respect to the dying.
4. To support family members.
5. Ensure good coordination of care.

To meet these needs, we must be aware of not only individual interpretations of such but also cultural interpretations. Although western medicine dictates that individuals should be fully informed and aware of their conditions, within Asian cultures for example to inform individuals of the life shortening nature of their condition is not advised and perceived as an act against beneficence (Searight and Gaford, 2005). This is also found within Latin cultures. In addition, both Asian and Latin cultures operationalise family decision-making as a priority over individual decision making, especially if there are talks to be held over life support options (Blackhall et al., 1995). More detailed discussion of truth telling, and concealment can be found in Chapter 4.

Individuals with neurodegenerative conditions

Despite the philosophy of palliative care being focused upon resolving pain and suffering, many studies detail how individuals can still sometimes die in pain (Steinhauser et al., 2002). There is a wealth of studies that further identify how a high proportion of individuals with neurodegeneration as compared to other disease groups, may die with pain undiagnosed and untreated (Barber and Murphy, 2011). In acknowledging this evidence base, health and social care professionals must begin to take a lead in discussing care planning and specifically advanced care planning early with families to ensure that the child or young person receive optimum cares and that their end-of-life care wishes transcend. Advance care planning promotes shared decision making and allows individuals and families to have the time to think about difficult issues that may occur later in the disease trajectory. For example, preferred place of death, and if with advanced illness they would want tube feeding to commence and if there should be artificial hydration or not.

Children's understandings of death and dying

Understanding death and embracing end of life care is a complex and emotional process for families. For children and young people their understanding is determined by their appreciation of the following facts:

1. All humans eventually die (inevitability),
2. All living species eventually die (universality),
3. Death is final, it is not reversible (irreversibility),
4. Death means that all our bodily functions stop working (cessation), and
5. Death itself is resultant of bodily processes closing down (causality) (Jaakkola and Slaughter, 2002).

Understanding of these facts is reached by children at different ages but we can be guided in practice by the developmental psychology literature that has evaluated at what developmental stages children can begin to understand.

At five years children can start to appreciate inevitability and universality. However, their understanding of universality and cessation can take them to being nearer to seven years of age. There have been studies that also identify that once children start to appreciate cessation, it can take them longer to accept that thinking processes and emotionality also cease when physical body processes do (Panagiotaki et al., 2015). This can relate to family spiritual and religious belief systems and can lead to children having supernatural beliefs about death (Lane et al., 2016).

A few interesting studies have been conducted in diverse cultures across the world about children and adult death beliefs. In Madagascar, people believe that their deceased ancestors are still present amongst the living (Astuti and Harris, 2008). This finding was also evident in Tanna, Vanatu, a Melanesian archipelago (Watson-Jones et al., 2017). These studies and others identify that there are some cross-cultural similarities in death belief systems:

1. Children are more likely to continue to believe that psychological processes such as dreaming continue beyond bodily death. This is not unique to children though, because many adults have held on to this belief too.

2. The scientific explanation of death and the more supernatural ones that can relate to spiritual and religious belief systems can co-exist for children and adults alike without conflicts.
3. This dual thinking process is not reflective of age or developmental stage because once scientific knowledge of death is understood the alternative belief system continues (Astuti and Harris, 2008; Watson-Jones et al., 2017).

Lane et al. (2016) has also suggested from exploring the death beliefs of religious American children compared to nonreligious Chinese children, that the dual belief system of scientific and supernatural death beliefs is more prevalent in individuals from religious cultures. The influence of afterlife beliefs on psychological functioning at the end of life is of interest to palliative care professionals. McClain-Jacobson et al. (2004) conducted a systematic analysis of afterlife beliefs in individuals receiving end of life care. Their results highlighted lower levels of end-of-life despair (hopelessness, desire for hastened death and suicidal ideation) in individuals who held a belief in an afterlife compared to participants unsure or who did not hold such beliefs.

The unspeakable nature of childhood death and dying

While scholars debate the 'good death,' death and dying for children and young people and their families is often considered to be a topic that is too difficult to talk about. Death and dying in children and young people remain to be a silent phenomenon. As a result, there is a reflective gap in the literature surrounding what may constitute a good death for a child or young person with a serious illness. This gap is concerning because children and young people do live with serious illness, anticipatory grief, and death and do want to understand what is happening to them and to have their worries relieved. Silencing discussions is often made on developmental grounds but can heighten fear around death and dying for children and young people and their families. This is despite evidence that has shown parents have felt better when conversations have been had with their children about dying (Bates and Kearney, 2015).

We also have evidence that children often will have awareness that they are dying, even when there has not been any conversation between themselves and their families or caregivers about it (Bluebond-Langner, 1978/2020). The lack of parental and societal acceptance to talk about these matters with children and young people is understandable, However, where there is a lack of acceptance this establishes an unspeakable nature to the phenomenon. This silence undermines the possibility of personal acceptance on the part of the child or young person. The silence plays a dual role to not talk about something that is feared and to perpetuate the stigma which can also prevent meaningful conversations in the clinical setting. Even in conversations about the death of a loved one, children and young people can often be protected from witnessing the end-of-life phase or be involved in funerals. They are aware that death is being kept as a secret from them and can lead to 'death ambivalence' (Paul, 2019).

Developmental psychologists have to some degree also helped this perpetuation of silence in suggesting children comprehend death differently through their stages of cognitive development, suggesting some children unable to process the complexity of their condition, never mind their life shortening prognosis (Brand et al., 2017). Therefore, silence in relation to childhood death arises for clinical, social and theoretical reasons. However, the mainstream developmental theories and adult persuasions to keep things secret do not acknowledge the social constructionist work on universal childhood experiences. In diverse cultural and social contexts, children and young people can have diverse perspectives and capacities. To this end, there are children and young people, from even at a very young age who can comprehend death and dying and would benefit from related conversations (Stern, 1985).

When it comes to understanding the capacities of a child to engage in conversations around death and dying, whether related to their own condition or that of a loved one, it is encouraged that health and social care professionals and families employ an independent case approach. To not assume child or young person capacity or to use a general approach. The approach needs to be considerate of each individual, what they may already know and understand and what they desire to know, in collaboration with the family.

The death positivity movement

In recent years we have seen the onset and development of the death positivity movement. The movement was inspired by the prize winning anthropological work of Ernest Becker's (1973), The Denial of Death. The death-positive movement aims to inspire open conversations about death and dying for all, regardless of people's belief and value systems. This is to disrupt the culture of silence that exists around these topics. Death-positivity groups, for example, The Order of the Good Death (2021) first established in the USA by Caitlin Doughty, and Dying Matters, a campaign associated with Hospices UK (Dying Matters, 2022), each aim to bring death and dying conversations into the public discourse.

The death-positive movement has also given rise to more open discussions about death in the general media – for example, the podcast Griefcast, hosted by Cariad Lloyd, and the annual Good Grief festival (2021), a virtual festival exploring the themes of attachment and loss. This body of work encourages all aspects of death and dying to be explored. Working in a collaborative way, the primary intention is to engage members of the public, inspire and empower them to talk openly about death and dying, to be informed and to make plans. If the good death is one of awareness and informational provision, then this movement is of instrumental support to it.

Facing death

No matter how young people may plan and try to be prepared for their end-of-life care. The realities of that experience can be fraught with emotional difficulties. In the academic literature we do not have a depth of material to glean the child or young person's experience beyond more physiological or medical papers detailing death process and symptomology. The children and young person's palliative care evidence base continues to lack the voice of the individual experiencing serious illness. However, we can infer theoretical relevance to stories and recounts of experiences via people documenting their experiences outside of the academic and professional literature base.

Dame Deborah James, fondly known as the social media influencer and media writer, the 'Bowel babe' is one shining example of how a young person with serious illness can influence a culture to become more aware of the symptoms of serious illness, the impacts on day to day lives, living life to the fullest and the realities of facing death and dying in their end-of-life care.

Over the weekend of the late Queen Elizabeth's jubilee celebrations, just a week following Deborah's announcement that she was at the end of her life, Deborah engaged in a telephone conversation with her friend and fellow writer, Lizzie Parry (3 June 2022). She reflected on her final days with her family. Her words give us some sense of what dying was like for Deborah, her words can also connect readers with some key messages relative to 'dying well':

> *There's no right or wrong way to die, I'm still doing this my way. I'm frustrated with my situation because I don't want to die. I don't think I will ever really accept it. I was given days, to a week, to live when I left the hospital. But I'm still here. I don't really believe that it's happening. It all feels like a horrible joke. Watching the demise of my body is really, really sad...I was someone who, even for most of my time living with cancer, was fit and healthy. So to see myself like this now, it's heart breaking.*

The disbelief and denial of death is an emotion theorised in the work of Kubler Ross and others who have explored the dying experiences of individuals and their anticipatory and lived through grieving for their impeding death, loss of self and family. Mastery over one's death is as important as mastery over one's illness and related quality of life outcomes for many individuals with serious illness. Children and young people's palliative care and its ethos of person and family centred care, shared, advanced and supported decision-making processes, tries to ensure that the individual's values and wishes are at the centre of all cares and support. Research has indicated that where individuals can maintain a level of control over their lives there are better psychological wellbeing outcomes for them and their families. However, this does not mean that even with the best care, that when individuals are close to their death that they will not be sad or experience distress. It is recognised that dying is a complex process, but it is hoped that where individuals are supported to complete life goals throughout their illness, and can complete final wishes, then there is the possibility that they can then feel more at peace as death becomes closer to their reach (Chochinov, 2012).

It is the work of palliative care professionals, families and others who can help to scaffold individuals dying wishes and experiences with compassion:

> *I've found I need a routine…Getting dressed every day is huge, it's an enormous source of strength for me. Putting on make-up is the same, I do it every day. I like looking like myself, it makes me feel better…People might look at me and think, 'Just spend time with your family'. They might question why I'm doing all this – the book launch, the T-shirts, raising money for my BowelBabe Fund. The truth is, it's giving me purpose in my final days. It's amazing what you can do with a deadline – the ultimate one. And my family are all a part of this with me. We're doing it our way.*
>
> *When I ask Debs what the hardest part of dying is – aside from leaving loved ones – she is as brutally honest as ever.*
>
> *It's the pressure to make memories… It's a really hard thing to do when you're dying… People say, 'Just enjoy time with your kids'. Of course, that's what I want to do but I feel exhausted, sick and in pain and I can't move, so it limits what you can do. Making memories is really, really hard when you don't have the physical capacity.*

As highlighted in the prologue to this book, people with serious illness have an array of coping strategies available to them, with advancing years they have learnt ways to cope with other issues. However, the coping over time moves more and more towards strategies that enable a positive outlook, a focus away from the illness itself and maintaining a sense of normality. Deborah modified her expectations but maintained a sense of normality through routine, a routine that was also serving to preserve her dignity. For Deborah, looking her best was spiritually meaningful, being still able to brush her own hair and put on her own lipstick was extremely important to her. And despite the level of her physical suffering, she strived to maintain her identity and purpose as a mother, actively engaging in memory making. Her focus on maintaining purpose also met with her public identity and she continued to build her legacy in this area of her life too. Deborah's need for generativity was visible and this also served to promote her dignity, maintaining her poise, for her family and followers.

The care and support of Deborah's family was strong. Through her scaffold of support Deborah harnessed growth through her trauma; her sibling bonds strengthened, and her sibling relationships became increasingly valued. The experience showed her how much they cared, indeed there was a mutuality of care and compassion. For Deborah, the deepening of bonds, is what appeared to be one aspect of the silver lining of the experience for her.

> *There's no blueprint to how you're going to feel when you're dying. Emotions change, second by second, hour by hour. I'm scared because I don't know what to expect. It's a really scary thing to face, I'm only 40, and it's heartbreaking knowing what I am*

> *leaving behind. What's really hard is that no one talks about death, we don't really know what happens or how we're meant to navigate it. Death is life's last taboo. I hope that by talking about it a bit, I might bring some comfort to others.*
>
> *I understand now why animals take themselves off to die. No one can fix me. Everyone has an opinion on what I should do, whether I should take these drugs or not. It's because they care – it's all out of love and nobody wants to see me in pain. It must be as painful for them as it is for me. This is happening to them too.*

Through serious illness comes many challenges, the greatest of all is perhaps living through the final weeks and days toward death if there remains the awareness of the body struggling but the mind still is wanting to continue to embrace life. We have no template on how to live with a serious illness, just as we have no template on how to die, no checklist. For an individual who has managed so well to maintain control and autonomy through their illness, this lack of direction to assist decision making in a period of unknowingness and high uncertainty, can be overwhelming. Uncertainty is a difficult challenge for all individuals with serious illness and their families and can arrive at different junctures.

An acceptance that people may want different experiences toward the end of their lives is a philosophy to be promoted across professional, family and community boundaries. Dying people will struggle intensely on both a physical and emotional level, they might not always make sense, because saying goodbye is difficult. As noted, serious illness can be a great biographical disruption, or a journey of small disruptions, an oscillation of normalisation and trauma that can also include periods of biographical suspension. In Deborah's words we can interpret that perhaps dying people also mentally suspend their dying, to normalise their everyday, to focus on the present, the memory making and living life to the fullest, to cope. Once the death draws nearer the suspension ends, and the normalisation is too difficult to maintain and grapple with. It is now mostly biographical disruption, and it takes great inner strength to keep positive, if only for loved ones. Removing the taboos, the silence, and allowing sharing, has the potential to promote 'dying well', a 'good' or perhaps a 'better' death.

Funerals

Death is the final life transition, the funeral is the rite of passage for the dead and the living, assisting the bereaved and enabling the death to be further conceptualised as 'socially good.' Indeed, funeral rites are considered to have three distinct functions to concretise the good death transition. Funerals allow the respectful disposal of the body, they also:

1. Provide psychological care to the bereaved, reasoning and regulating new identities and relationships resultant of the death.
2. Assist the transference of the deceased from this world and into the next.

3. Provide an outlet for which the bereaved can deal with their grief and for some also their guilt. The acting out of grief in the presence of a captive and empathic support group can enhance wellbeing and positive reflections on the good life and death of the deceased.

The nature of funerals can be dependent on the age of the deceased. The lives of older adults are more likely to be celebrated. The mood of a child's funeral is quite different and with every anniversary the deceased can be mentally resurrected in memorial. As noted briefly already, death, funeral and burial rituals vary across cultures. However, all funerals transition the identity of the deceased to a dead person. In some cultures, the dead can also take on board a new identity of ancestor and as someone who will remain a part of the family or as a soul that although returning to be in the company of God will remain watchful over their families. In contrast, the Achuar of eastern Ecuador are encouraged to forget the deceased. They believe dead people want to take revenge on the living and so will want to maintain a vengeful presence. They believe harm could come to the living if connections are maintained, therefore much ritual is performed to eliminate bonds.

Regardless of belief systems and the nature of rituals, funerals mark the beginning on new lives. For example, a life as a widow or a life as the head of the family. The role transformation is a time boundless process for most, as it can take time to adjust to new identities, for some it can take a lifetime (Eisma et al., 2022).

Chapter summary

We all strive for the 'good' death, one that is constructed as such in personally and socially meaningful terms. In western societies the 'good' death where possible is couched in a world of truth telling and one that has allowed autonomous decision making for both individuals and families. Guidance and ritual that draw on spiritual and religious belief systems and practices can be drawn upon to make the dying process, death, and funeral processes honourable. Irrespective of condition advanced planning can also assist wellbeing toward the end of life. In the example of individuals with conditions that can degenerate capacity, it is especially important to allow individuals and families the time to plan. For children, the difficult task of caring and of anticipating and saying goodbye can be so much harder for families. The child's understanding of death can be compounded by their age and developmental state and their previous experiences. For many families, the burden of care can be immense, and they need support to then consider more open conversations with children and young people about death and dying.

Overall, end-of-life care is an ongoing, dynamic process involving the interplay of health and social care professionals, individuals, and families that is moderated by spirituality, culture, and personal preferences (among other factors). Professionals should therefore not assume but ask about individual preferences and needs from the point of entry into the palliative care world and engage with wider communities in supporting individuals through to their death. More work is needed to promote social acceptance of dying well, because death happens to us all and is perceived as 'good' from both private and social horizons.

Key issues

1. There is no universally shared definition of bodily death. There is definitional debate around biomedical death and cultural differences exist with respect to death and the transcendence of spirit or soul.
2. There exists an element of death anxiety in all cultures. It is the role of palliative care to support end of life wishes and to alleviate existential suffering, so that individuals can hopefully end their lives in peace.
3. Where there is scope, a 'good death' or 'dying well' can be facilitated by end-of-life care planning and other tailored interventions that support challenging conversations, meaning making and legacy leaving. This can ease individual and family burden in the longer term.
4. Professional appreciation of the spiritual and religious belief systems and related needs of individuals and families in their care can facilitate death ritual and further meet end of life wishes.
5. The notion of the 'good death' is a historical concept that has evolved from supported dying. Although we may now use different terminology in practice, there remains individual, familial and cultural perceptions around what the good death or dying well may constitute for individuals.
6. Post death rituals and funerals ease family suffering.

Box 7.1 Reflective questions

1. Can you relate to the historical conception of a 'good death'? Is this concept still relevant for children, young people and families?
2. How do you perceive a 'good' death? (What experiences influence your perception?)
3. What death rituals does your culture use to support 'dying well'? (Are they like those used by your peers/colleagues?)

References

Abu-Ras, W. and Laird, L., 2011. How Muslim and non-Muslim chaplains serve Muslim patients? Does the interfaith chaplaincy model have room for Muslims' experiences? *Journal of religion and Health*, *50*(1), pp.46–61.

An, E., 2018. *Death-related Distress in Advanced Cancer* (Doctoral dissertation, University of Toronto (Canada)).

Astuti, R. and Harris, P.L., 2008. Understanding mortality and the life of the ancestors in rural Madagascar. *Cognitive Science*, *32*(4), pp.713–740.

Barber, J. and Murphy, K., 2011. Challenges that specialist palliative care nurses encounter when caring for patients with advanced dementia. *International Journal of Palliative Nursing*, *17*(12), pp.587–591.

Bates, A.T. and Kearney, J.A., 2015. Understanding death with limited experience in life: dying children's and adolescents' understanding of their own terminal illness and death. *Current Opinion in Supportive and Palliative Care*, *9*(1), p.40.

Bauer-Wu, S., Barrett, R. and Yeager, K., 2007. Spiritual perspectives and practices at the end-of-life: A review of the major world religions and application to palliative care. *Indian Journal of Palliative Care*, *13*(2), p.53.

Becker, E. 1973. *The Denial of Death.* The Free Press New York.

Beckstrand, R.L., Callister, L.C. and Kirchhoff, K.T., 2006. Providing a 'good death': critical care nurses' suggestions for improving end-of-life care. *American Journal of Critical Care*, *15*(1), pp.38–45.

Blackhall, L.J., Murphy, S.T., Frank, G., Michel, V. and Azen, S., 1995. Ethnicity and attitudes toward patient autonomy. *Jama*, *274*(10), pp.820–825.

Bluebond-Langner, M., 1978/2020. The private worlds of dying children. In *The Private Worlds of Dying Children.* Princeton University Press.

Brand, S., Wolfe, J. and Samsel, C., 2017. The impact of cancer and its treatment on the growth and development of the pediatric patient. *Current pediatric reviews*, *13*(1), pp.24–33.

Braun, K.L. and Zir, A., 2001. Roles for the church in improving end-of-life care: Perceptions of Christian clergy and laity. *Death Studies*, *25*(8), pp.685–704.

Brennan, M. and Letherby, G., 2017. Auto/biographical approaches to researching death and bereavement: Connections, continuums, contrasts. *Mortality*, *22*(2), pp.155–169.

Burke, B.L., Martens, A. and Faucher, E.H., 2010. Two decades of terror management theory: A meta-analysis of mortality salience research. *Personality and Social Psychology Review*, *14*(2), pp.155–195.

Burns, J.P. and Mitchell, C., 2005. Is there any consensus about end-of-life care in pediatrics?. *Archives of Pediatrics & Adolescent Medicine*, *159*(9), pp.889–891.

Busch, J.T., Watson-Jones, R.E. and Legare, C.H., 2020. Cultural variation in the development of beliefs about conservation. *Cognitive Science*, *44*(10), p.e12909.

Chochinov, H.M., 2012. *Dignity therapy: final words for final days.* OUP USA.

de Beauvoir S., 1966. *A Very Easy Death.* O'Brian P, trans. New York, NY: GP Putnam Sons.

Depaola, S.J., Griffin, M., Young, J.R. and Neimeyer, R.A., 2003. Death anxiety and attitudes towardthe elderly among older adults: The Role of gender and ethnicity. *Death Studies*, *27*(4), pp.335–354.

Downey, L., Curtis, J.R., Lafferty, W.E., Herting, J.R. and Engelberg, R.A., 2010. The Quality of Dying and Death Questionnaire (QODD): empirical domains and theoretical perspectives. *Journal of pain and symptom management*, *39*(1), pp.9–22.

Duff, R.W. and Hong, L.K., 1995. Age density, religiosity and death anxiety in retirement communities. *Review of Religious Research*, pp.19–32.

Dying Matters, Hospice UK, 2021. www.hospiceuk.org/our-campaigns/dying-matters (accessed 20 May 2022)

Dying Matters, Hospice UK, 2022. www.hospiceuk.org/our-campaigns/dying-matters (Accessed 14 December 2022).

Eisma, M.C., de Lang, T.A. and Stroebe, M.S., 2022. Restoration-oriented stressors of bereavement. *Anxiety, Stress, & Coping*, *35*(3), pp.339–353.

Field, D., 1996. Awareness and modern dying. *Mortality*, *1*(3), pp.255–265.

Flueckiger, J.B., 2006. *In Amma's Healing Room: Gender and Vernacular Islam in South India.* Indiana University Press.

Gardiner, D., Shemie, S., Manara, A. and Opdam, H., 2012. International perspective on the diagnosis of death. *British journal of anaesthesia*, *108*(suppl_1), pp.i14-i28.

Gatrad, A.R., 1994. Muslim customs surrounding death, bereavement, postmortem examinations, and organ transplants. *BMJ*, *309*(6953), pp.521–523.

Gatrad, R. and Sheikh, A., 2002. Palliative care for Muslims and issues after death. *International Journal of Palliative Nursing*, *8*(12), pp.594–597.

Gazelle, G., 2003. A good death: not just an abstract concept. *Journal of Clinical Oncology: Official Journal of the American Society of Clinical Oncology*, *21*(9 Suppl), pp.95s–96s.

Glaser, B.G. and Strauss, A.L., 2017. *Time for Dying*. Routledge.

Good grief festival, 2021., https://goodgrieffest.com/ (accessed 20 May 2022).

Griefcast, hosted by Cariad Lloyd, 2022. https://cariadlloyd.com/griefcast (accessed 20 May 2022)

Gyatso, T. (the XIV Dalai Lama) and Jinpa, T., 1995. The world of Tibetan Buddhism: An overview of its philosophy and practice. Wisdom Publications

Hales, S., Chiu, A., Husain, A., Braun, M., Rydall, A., Gagliese, L., Zimmermann, C. and Rodin, G., 2014. The quality of dying and death in cancer and its relationship to palliative care and place of death. *Journal of Pain and Symptom Management*, *48*(5), pp.839–851.

Hartford Foundation, 2016. Conversation stopper What's preventing physicians from talking with patients about end-of-life and advance care planning. www.johnahartford.org/newsroom/view/national-poll-conversation-stopper-whats-preventing-physicians-from-talking/ (accessed 15 May 2022).

Hertogh, C.M., 2006. Advance care planning and the relevance of a palliative care approach in dementia. *Age and Ageing*, *35*(6), pp.553–555.

Hoelter, J.W., 1979. Multidimensional treatment of fear of death. *Journal of Consulting and Clinical Psychology*, *47*(5), p.996.

Jaakkola, R.O. and Slaughter, V., 2002. Children's body knowledge: Understanding 'life' as a biological goal. *British Journal of Developmental Psychology*, *20*(3), pp.325–342.

Joint Royal Colleges Ambulance Liaison Committee, 2019. *JRCALC clinical guidelines 2019*. Class Professional Publishing.

Kastenbaum, R., 2000. *The Psychology of Death*. Springer Publishing Company.

Kawano, S., 2011. A sociocultural analysis of death anxiety among older Japanese urbanites in a citizens' movement. *OMEGA-Journal of Death and Dying*, *62*(4), pp.369–386.

Kearl, M.C., 1996. Dying well: The unspoken dimension of aging well. *American Behavioral Scientist*, *39*(3), pp.336–360.

Kellehear, A., 1990. *Dying of Cancer: The Final Year of Life*. Taylor & Francis US.

Kissane, D.W., 2014. Demoralization: a life-preserving diagnosis to make for the severely medically ill. *Journal of Palliative Care*, *30*(4), pp.255–258.

Kramer, K., 1988. *The Sacred Art of Dying: How World Religions Understand Death.* Paulist Press.

Lane, J.D., Zhu, L., Evans, E.M. and Wellman, H.M., 2016. Developing concepts of the mind, body, and afterlife: Exploring the roles of narrative context and culture. *Journal of Cognition and Culture, 16*(1–2), pp.50–82.

Langer, R., 2007. *Buddhist Rituals of Death and Rebirth: Contemporary Sri Lankan Practice and its Origins.* Routledge.

Mack, J.W., Cronin, A., Keating, N.L., Taback, N., Huskamp, H.A., Malin, J.L., Earle, C.C. and Weeks, J.C., 2012. Associations between end-of-life discussion characteristics and care received near death: a prospective cohort study. *Journal of Clinical Oncology, 30*(35), p.4387.

McClain-Jacobson, C., Rosenfeld, B., Kosinski, A., Pessin, H., Cimino, J.E. and Breitbart, W., 2004. Belief in an afterlife, spiritual well-being and end-of-life despair in patients with advanced cancer. *General hospital psychiatry, 26*(6), pp.484–486.

McNamara, B., 2004. Good enough death: autonomy and choice in Australian palliative care. *Social Science & Medicine, 58*(5), pp.929–938.

McNamara, B., Waddell, C. and Colvin, M., 1995. Threats to the good death: the cultural context of stress and coping among hospice nurses. *Sociology of Health & Illness, 17*(2), pp.222–241.

Meier, E.A., Gallegos, J.V., Thomas, L.P.M., Depp, C.A., Irwin, S.A. and Jeste, D.V., 2016. Defining a good death (successful dying): literature review and a call for research and public dialogue. *The American Journal of Geriatric Psychiatry, 24*(4), pp.261–271.

Neimeyer, R.A., and Moore, M.K., 1994. Validity and reliability of the Multidimensional Fear of Death Scale. In R. A. Neimeyer (Ed.), *Death Anxiety Handbook: Research, Instrumentation, and Application* (pp. 103–119). Taylor & Francis

Panagiotaki, G., Nobes, G., Ashraf, A. and Aubby, H., 2015. British and Pakistani children's understanding of death: Cultural and developmental influences. *British Journal of Developmental Psychology, 33*(1), pp.31–44.

Parry, L., 2022. *HER FINAL DAYS I'm being a b*tch because I'm so angry I'm dying – I don't want friends to see me this way, says Dame Deborah James.* The Sun. 3 June. www.thesun.co.uk/health/18775829/dame-deborah-james-angry-dying/ (accessed 3 June 2022).

Parsuram, A. and Sharma, M., 1992. Functional relevance of belief in life-after-death. *Journal of Personality and Clinical Studies, 8*(1–2), 97–100.

Paul, S., 2019. Is death taboo for children? Developing death ambivalence as a theoretical framework to understand children's relationship with death, dying and bereavement. *Children & Society, 33*(6), pp.556–571.

President's Commission for the Study of Ethical Problems in Medicine, Biomedical, and Behavioral Research. 1981. *Protecting human subjects: first biennial report on the adequacy and uniformity of federal rules and policies, and their implementation, for the protection of human subjects in biomedical and behavioral research.* Washington, DC: President's Commission for the Study of Ethical Problems in Medicine, Biomedical, and Behavioral Research.

Pyszczynski, T., Solomon, S. and Greenberg, J., 2015. Thirty years of terror management theory: From genesis to revelation. In *Advances in Experimental Social Psychology* (Vol. 52, pp. 1–70). Academic Press.

Rodriguez, A. and King, N., 2014. Sharing the care: the key-working experiences of professionals and the parents of life-limited children. *International Journal of Palliative Nursing*, *20*(4), pp.165–171.

Rosenblatt, P.C., 2008. Grief across cultures: A review and research agenda. In M. S. Stroebe, R. O. Hansson, H. Schut, & W. Stroebe (Eds.), *Handbook of bereavement research and practice: Advances in theory and intervention* (pp. 207–222). American Psychological Association

Schumaker, J.F., Barraclough, R.A. and Vagg, L.M., 1988. Death anxiety in Malaysian and Australian university students. *The Journal of Social Psychology*, *128*(1), pp.41–47.

Seale, C., 1998. Constructing death: The sociology of dying and bereavement. Cambridge University Press.

Searight, H.R. and Gafford, J., 2005. Cultural diversity at the end of life: issues and guidelines for family physicians. *American Family Physician*, *71*(3), pp.515–522.

Singer, P.A., Martin, D.K. and Kelner, M., 1999. Quality end-of-life care: patients' perspectives. *Jama*, *281*(2), pp.163–168.

Steinhauser, K.E., Bosworth, H.B., Clipp, E.C., McNeilly, M., Christakis, N.A., Parker, J. and Tulsky, J.A., 2002. Initial assessment of a new instrument to measure quality of life at the end of life. *Journal of Palliative Medicine*, *5*(6), pp.829–841.

Steinhauser, K.E., Clipp, E.C., McNeilly, M., Christakis, N.A., McIntyre, L.M. and Tulsky, J.A., 2000. In search of a good death: observations of patients, families, and providers. *Annals of Internal Medicine*, *132*(10), pp.825–832.

Stern, E.M., 1985. *Psychotherapy and the Grieving Patient*. Psychology Press.

Tam, K.P., 2013. Existential motive underlying cosmetic surgery: A terror management analysis. *Journal of Applied Social Psychology*, *43*(5), pp.947–955.

Tapsfield, A., 2006. Improving the care of dying patients in the community. *Nursing Times*, *102*(35), pp.28–30.

Teno, J.M., Clarridge, B.R., Casey, V., Welch, L.C., Wetle, T., Shield, R. and Mor, V., 2004. Family perspectives on end-of-life care at the last place of care. *Jama*, *291*(1), pp.88–93.

The End-of-Life Care Strategy (2008) www.gov.uk/government/publications/end-of-life-care-strategy-promoting-high-quality-care-for-adults-at-the-end-of-their-life (accessed 10 May 2022).

The Order of the Good Death, 2021. www.orderofthegooddeath.com/our-story/ (accessed 16 May 2022).

The President's Commission for the Study of Ethical Problems in Medicine and Biomedical and Behavioural Research, Abram, M.B., 1981. *Defining Death: A Report on the Medical, Legal and Ethical Issues in the Determination of Death*. The Commission.

Together for Short Lives, 2012. guidance for children's end of life care www.togetherforshortlives.org.uk/resource/guide-end-life-care/ (accessed 10 May 2022).

Truog, R., 2004. Brain death: at once 'well settled' and 'persistently unresolved'. *AMA Journal of Ethics*, *6*(8), pp.357–359.

Truog, R.D., Campbell, M.L., Curtis, J.R., Haas, C.E., Luce, J.M., Rubenfeld, G.D., Rushton, C.H. and Kaufman, D.C., 2008. Recommendations for end-of-life care in the intensive care unit: a consensus statement by the American College of Critical Care Medicine. *Critical care medicine*, *36*(3), pp.953–963.

Watson-Jones, R.E., Busch, J.T., Harris, P.L. and Legare, C.H., 2017. Does the body survive death? Cultural variation in beliefs about life everlasting. *Cognitive Science*, *41*, pp.455–476.

Weisman, A.D., 1972. *On Dying and Denying: A Psychiatric Study of Terminality*. Behavioural Publications.
Wiener, L., Bedoya, S., Battles, H., Sender, L., Zabokrtsky, K., Donovan, K.A., Thompson, L.M., Di Ciccone, B.B.L., Babilonia, M.B., Fasciano, K. and Malinowski, P., 2022. Voicing their choices: advance care planning with adolescents and young adults with cancer and other serious conditions. *Palliative & Supportive Care*, *20*(4), pp.462–470.
Zaslow, J. and Pausch, R., 2014. *The Last Lecture*. Hyperion.

8 Grief and bereavement in children, young people, and families

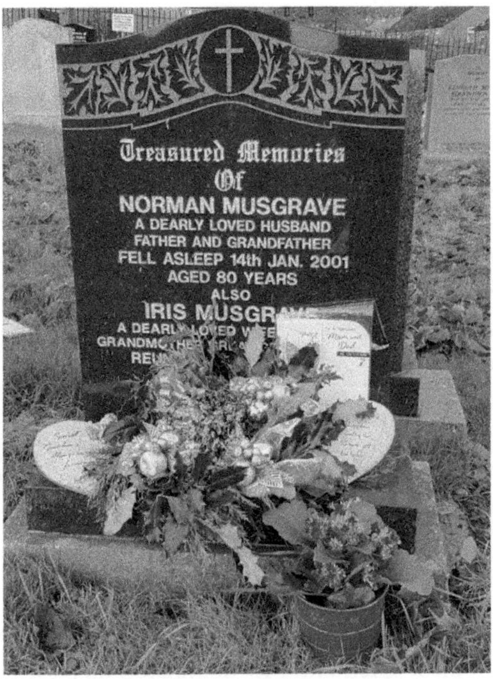
Treasured Memories
Of
NORMAN MUSGRAVE
A DEARLY LOVED HUSBAND
FATHER AND GRANDFATHER
FELL ASLEEP 14th JAN. 2001
AGED 80 YEARS
ALSO

Figure 8.1 A photograph of a loved one's grave.
Photograph taken by Alison Rodriguez.

Introduction

When our loved ones die, we find ourselves in a place of bereavement, a state of loss (Attig, 2012). Bereavement disrupts the rhythm of our everyday lives as we experience the sorrow of grief and its emotional, psychological, cognitive, physical, and spiritual impacts (Zisook et al., 2010). The associated mourning

DOI: 10.4324/9781003340287-9

represents the culturally accepted expression of the personal feelings when bereaved. Diverse cultures hold different expectations of how we should behave following loss (Kubler-Ross and Kessler, 2005).

The length of public grief may be stipulated by some cultures, others there are demands in terms of outward appearance. For example, hair may have to be cut to symbolise the bereavement or you may have to wear black dress. In some cultures, death signifies a time for celebration so there will be music and dance and yet in other cultures demands will be more sombre and kinship may have to play out death rituals for the remainder of their existence (Rosenblatt, 2008). Although there are these quite diverse cultural practices, there are global similarities. In response to a death the emotions of fear, anger and upset signified by tears are commonplace and, in most cultures, this outward show of grief is acceptable behaviour (Parkes et al., 1997).

Health and social care professionals in palliative care help families cope with dying and bereavement. Their support is influenced by experience and influential grief theory. This chapter considers the loss of different relatives, how theory informs collective understandings, what is considered a normative response to grief and how responses can sometimes be pathologised. Grief is a major stressor, where deaths are expected, and where support is provided for anticipatory grieving, then there can be better outcomes for families. Often meaning reconstruction interventions are helpful and increasingly recognised as useful in bereavement support practices.

Contemporary grief theory

There are a multitude of grief theories that have evolved over the years, each drawing on different psychological perspectives, be they attachment, cognitive, psychodynamic, or general life-event situated (Stroebe and Archer, 2013; Stroebe et al., 2010).

Freudian conceptions

The article entitled 'Mourning and melancholia' authored by Freud (1917/1957) is the original theorisation of grief, one that dominated medical intervention for over fifty years. In Freud's articulation of 'grief work' the survivor engages in a process of breaking down the emotional connections they have had with the deceased. There are three parts to this process:

1. Cutting ties to the bereaved
2. Reorienting oneself to a new life without the deceased; and
3. Developing new relationships.

The grief work process involves strong emotions of guilt and anger. But if the separation is not acknowledged and the grief work not fully processed, then the grief itself can become complex and both mental and physical illness can ensue. This model of grief work promotes a 'moving on' to be able to return to a 'normal' level of functioning. Freud also suggested that normative reactions to grief should be short lived. However, he later acknowledged that his own experience of being bereaved of his daughter continued more than thirty years following her death. As such, in other writing's he empathises that the loss of a child is so great that grief can be long term with a desire for a continued bond with the child rather than a 'letting go' (Shapiro, 2001).

Seventeen years ago, Valentine's (2006) review of academic constructions of bereavement continued to identify Freudian language around dealing with grief, such as 'moving on' and 'letting go'. Psychological interventions continue to be aimed at helping individuals 'recover' and have been developed from the fixed, sequential, stage-like models whereby the final stage is acceptance. As Valentine (2006) poignantly states *'A normal, though painful part of life has become a condition that needs treating'* (p. 59).

Kubler-Ross

There was little attention given to grief and bereavement by social scientists until Elizabeth Kubler-Ross published her work 'On Death and Dying' in 1969 (Kubler-Ross, 1969). This book was instrumental in bringing the staged model of anticipatory grief into the public forum. Many professionals and the public have since continued to understand grief and bereavement as linear, and time bound. However, it is widely accepted that grief is complex, is subjective and experienced differently by different people. There may be times that these emotions identified by Kubler-Ross are relevant and experienced, but not always will they be experienced in a linear fashion. It is argued that coping with dying is a richer and more complex process than merely progressing through certain ill-defined stages. Indeed, Kubler-Ross herself in her opening paragraph of 'On Grief and Grieving' (Kessler, 2004 p1) states:

> *The stages have evolved since their introduction, and they have been very misunderstood over the past three decades. They were never meant to help tuck messy emotions into packages. They are responses to loss that many people have, but there is not a typical response to loss, as there is no typical loss. Our grief is as individual as our lives. Not everyone goes through all of them or goes in a prescribed order.*

Still, stage theories are appealing to those working in both research and practice – they allure us to consider a grief trajectory or order of events that we can observe until a person's grief is completed. Many positivist researchers also like to categorise grief so they can relate to 'at risk' factors and compute multidimensional models.

Where models are developed, they are interpreted in practice as indicators of norms. These can then be adopted in nonreflexive ways, which can mean complex experiences are missed. Yet, it is hard to see how the unique experience of bereavement can in any way be conceptualised (Hale, 1996).

In general, studies of grief and bereavement have not been able to identify any clear patterns to 'normative' grieving. Individuals and families can differently interpret any level of adaptation. Some people suggest that the loss of certain loved ones is never adapted to or recovered from, but individuals can continue to manage day to day life. This then makes any assumptions around unhealthy grieving difficult to substantiate. Applying models of grief that argue a normative process is linear or even time bound can be unhelpful. Individuals may begin to think they are doing the grieving wrong or that how they are feeling or reacting, is at risk of being pathologised. As such individuals can feel disempowered in their grief experience (Friedman and James, 2008). Encouraged by these criticisms, and supported by a contextualist, constructivist, and interpretive shift in psychology (Neimeyer, 1998; Neimeyer and Mahoney, 1996), a new stream of grief theories are slowly emerging. These are thought to reflect a changing 'zeitgeist' about the meaning of loss in human experience.

Bowlby and Murray Parkes

The work of British psychiatrists John Bowlby and Colin Murray Parkes around bereavement has been influential with respect to palliative care provision for children and young people and the hospice movement. They collaborated on studying the grief process in the 1980s, drawing on Bowlby's 'Attachment Theory' (1980) and Parkes' (1998) studies of human information processing. Their work also analysed Kübler-Ross's five stages of grief which they later reformulated into a four-phase grief process. They noted the phases were likely not to be linear and could be retriggered by experiences and anniversaries.

Firstly, shock and disbelief, replaces denial. They argue that this is the human response to cope with the immediate reality of loss. Humans react to the immediate stress by shutting down to protect themselves and only opening themselves to the reality of what has happened in small stages. The full reality of the situation is not immediately acknowledged. It is something that slowly is put into the full consciousness of the person leading the person to perhaps feel they need to withdraw to slowly adapt. They are likely to feel numb and unresponsive.

During the second phase of their model, *searching and yearning*, the person tries to reconsider the reality with thoughts such as 'This couldn't have happened!' 'Why us?' 'Why now?' The result of such is the person can become angry, also showing their upset.

In the third phase, the person moves into a situation of *disorganization and despair*, they begin to fully absorb the reality of the loss. Life has changed and with this extreme stress can follow a feeling that they too can longer go on. Depression can be present along with a level of dis-organisation, absentmindedness, and apathy.

These combined responses are normative and mirror separation distress. As such it is argued that such emotional and behavioural responses should not be pathologised.

The final phase of grief in this model is *rebuilding and healing*. The person will start to restructure and reconceptualise their lives, setting new goals. They begin to look forward. The grieving person will have a renewed sense of identity, which goes beyond the loss. The grieving person now can draw on more energy and become social again. They can start to view their grief and bereavement as an event in their life (Parkes, 1998).

Current dominant theories

The two most dominant grief theories of our current times are the Dual-Process Model (Stroebe and Schut, 1999) and the Task-Based Model (Worden, 2018). The Dual Process Model of Grief (Stroebe and Schut, 1999), is a psychological model of grief that has been developed from the literature on stress. It identifies grief as a process involving an individual's cognitive processing that transfers between two modes of functioning:

1. A loss orientation
2. A restoration orientation.

When the individual is in the loss orientation mode, they are engaged in emotion focused coping, feeling a spectrum of emotions in relation to the loss. Whereas when they are in the restoration orientation mode, they are in a state of active coping, instrumentally making life changes that will accommodate their loss and at times doing things that will take their mind away from dwelling on the painful emotion of the loss and focusing on the tasks that need to be completed to continue everyday functioning. The state the bereaved person is in will alter from one moment to the next, for example one day they may feel overcome with sadness and the next be able to go to work and concentrate on completing work tasks without any overt expression of loss. The state and time spent in each orientation will also be dependent on the characteristics of the individual and the culture they belong.

Worden (2018) also identified that grieving is not a static process and the bereaved move back and forth through different emotions. The task-based model, however, identifies that those who are bereaved engage in four tasks throughout their grieving experience:

1. Accepting the reality of the loss.
2. Processing the pain of grief.
3. Adjusting to life without the deceased (including both internal, external, and spiritual adjustments); and
4. Searching for an everlasting connection with the deceased whilst trying to live their new life.

In addition, there are seven factors relevant to us further understanding the individual's grief experience:

1. Who the deceased was
2. The nature of the relationship of the bereaved to the deceased
3. The mode of death
4. Historical antecedents
5. Personality variables
6. Social mediators; and
7. Co-existing stressors.

These determinants are dominant in the stress and wellbeing literature, conceptualised as risk and protective factors. They help us to understand the context of each person's grief experience. The nature and strength of the relationship the bereaved had with the deceased, their attachment style and if there were any ongoing conflicts with the deceased can each have important impacts on the grief experienced and expressed. Where the bereaved were at the time of death and the nature of the death can also influence their bereavement and grief experience. Certain types of deaths can 'disenfranchise' the bereaved (Doka, 2002). This can happen for a number of reasons; the mode of death is stigmatised, meaning it is difficult for it to be openly acknowledged or socially supported. This can still happen in some communities whereby the person died from suicide for example. Or because the loss does not fit nicely with social norms – so it could be that the relationship the deceased had with the bereaved was not openly accepted or because the person suffering the loss is being excluded from experiencing the loss. This can happen with children for example, if they are disallowed to attend funerals and embrace death rituals shared by others in their community. The loss of a friend, co-worker or neighbour can also be internalised as disenfranchised, because there is no socially recognised validation for the associated grief relevant to such relationships (Doka, 2008; Robson and Walter, 2013). It is often in these circumstances that individuals will internalise their grief to maintain their everyday functioning (Kauffman, 2011).

Everyone copes with grief differently; each individual and family has unique needs and faces different challenges. If we consider only stage theories to guide supportive cares, then we are unable to be considerate and empathetic towards individual and family needs.

Continuing bonds

The awareness of the unique nature of grief has altered our thinking about how successful grieving is resultant of the metaphorical letting go of the deceased. Instead, we can reconceptualise that successful grieving may involve both a letting go and a maintenance of bonds. Klass (2006) suggested that maintaining a connection with the deceased can be healthy. When bereaved, a person's life has ended but relationships with that person can continue. In this manner, although clearly no longer living, the deceased can remain to hold some presence in the bereaved person's life. A continuing bond in this respect is defined as *'the presence of an ongoing inner relationship with the deceased person by the bereaved individual'* (Stroebe and Schut, 2005).

Our humanness contends that the relationships and bonds we hold with people can be continuous and ever changing. We are experienced in accommodating changes in relationships. The deceased may become viewed as a role model, someone the bereaved can consider when decision making and reflecting on what directions to take in life (Klass, 1993; Russac et al., 2002). The continued bond may enable cognitive discussions with the deceased, to mentally talk through their grieving which can complement their religious or spiritual belief systems. The bereaved may have lucid dreams where they continue to experience the deceased or by engaging in death rituals such as grave visiting, they can feel comfort through the felt presence of the deceased. Often these continued bonds can be co-created with others by talking through beliefs and experiences (Field and Filanosky, 2010).

Historic studies discovered that at least half of the bereaved population report a sense of the presence of their deceased loved one (Datson and Marwit, 1997). It is hypothesised however, that this incidence is much greater but individuals fear conveying their experiences to others for fear of being labelled insane.

More recent literature has explored where continuing bonds can be helpful against when it is not. Field (2006) and Waugh et al. (2018) detail examples of continuing bonds that illuminate the bereaved struggle to accept the loss. This can happen when individuals refuse to accept that the loss has happened. Bowlby's (1980) early work also highlights that those with insecure attachment styles can be at risk of chronic or complex grief trajectories (Bonanno et al., 2004). The work of Field and Filanosky (2010) identifies that continued bonds with the deceased can be classified into two types: 'internalised' and 'externalised'. Internalised continued bonds are maintained through the bereaved maintaining cognitive relationship, mentally holding on to the relationship had and imagining how the deceased would respond or act to current situations and events that the bereaved person is living through. Externalised continued bonds are qualitatively different. The bereaved person will report feeling an actual physical closeness to the deceased, sometimes reporting they sensed their touch or visualised their presence. These experiences can also be conceptualised as delusional or be hallucinatory.

Where individuals are deemed to be suffering from complex grief experiences, there can be self-reported externalised continued bonds and poorer adjustment to life without their significant other.

Other scholars suggest that in addition to internalised and externalised continued bonds it is possible to experience a third type. Scholtes and Browne (2015) in researching the adaptive coping styles of parents bereaved of a child identified that 'transference' could be conceptualised as a type of continued bond. The process of transference is one that maintains a relationship with the deceased by honouring their wishes and maintaining their interests. This type of bond is a concrete expression of continuation and not hallucinatory or delusional. For example, a bereaved person may visit a grave to feel closer to the deceased, but they do not infer that whilst there that they also have a physical meeting with the deceased person.

In appreciating that these diverse types of continued bonds can be present and prevailing we are moving beyond historical grief and bereavement theories. We still, however, determine a normative and abnormal process of grieving based upon our conceptualisations of continued bonds. 'Unhealthy' continuing bonds are those whereby the bereaved has unresolved grief because they do not accept that the person is now dead. Their continuing bond expressions are relative to a desire to be in continued physical proximity to the deceased. Whereas the 'healthy' continued bonds are relevant to their new internalised relationships with the deceased. They are symbolic bonds that provide the bereaved with a greater acceptance of the loss.

The cultures and societies we are situated in also impact on the nature and duration of the continued bonds we hold with the deceased. In some cultures, an overt expression of grief is considered appropriate, in others the bereaved are discouraged from speaking with others about the deceased or their loss (Boerner and Heckhause, 2003). As such, there remains research to be conducted looking at when continuing bonds are useful and a hindrance to personal and social grieving processes. What constitutes expressions of continuing bonds also need further definition (Root and Exline, 2014). Some authors believe that our current understandings of continued bonds are too simplistic and the connections that are made to mental wellbeing and functioning are likely to be more complex (Field et al., 2008; Stroebe et al., 2010). As a result, Researchers ought to explore, using naturalistic methods of inquiry the nature and dominance of continued bond phenomena in different populations.

Age and loss

As highlighted in Chapter 7, there is still an acceptance in society to be closed about death and dying in the conversations we have with children and young people. The shared understanding is they do not understand, they will not cope. Children however, who are not given accurate information and do not have the awareness to work out the situation for themselves are prone to piecing together bits of information they have gleaned and then deriving interesting and false stories. If children and young people have been excluded from involvement with the person who has died through their dying process, it can then be difficult for them to accept the death. Children are always aware of the atmosphere around them even though they might pretend otherwise. We can identify that individuals and families may respond in diverse ways to death and bereavement, because of what they have already experienced in life, but also in relation to what developmental tasks they have completed. Our stage of development in terms of our biology, psychology, social context, and spirituality, is believed to impact to some extent on our death understandings and responses.

Infancy – When in infancy, the impact of the death of a main caregiver can have clear implications, more so if aged beyond six months (Coates and

Gaensbauer, 2009). Earlier, infants manage to cope if they are provided with constant care and nurturance. The effects on older infants can be observed through the disruption of sleep patterns and difficulties in self-soothing (Markese, 2013). Constant care and maintenance of routine can help the infant to adjust to their different world. In practice, the most instrumental support that can be provided is in supporting the remaining primary care giver to maintain supportive care of the infant.

Preschool children – preschool is a time of rapid maturation and a growth in independence and a time of learning to bond with figures outside of the immediate family context. As discussed in the previous chapter the permanency of death is not really grasped for most children until they are around seven years old. However, some children as young as two or three have shown a grasp of such. This can be related to their exposure to palliative care or other environments where they may have experienced loss of peers or family. Regardless of exposure and understanding, coping at this age appears to involve a dual functioning for most children. This involves rapid movements from short spells of tears to a return to longer durations of play.

Where parents or main caregivers are consistent with their empathy there is a lower risk of children later experiencing behavioural manifestations of the bereavement (Markese, 2013). Where therapeutic interventions have been directed at preschool children, they have not shown high levels of effectiveness (Currier et al., 2007). Naturalistic settings and opportunist conversational moments amidst the everyday routine allow for death talk that is deemed more useful and supportive. Direct communication is also preferred over fictitious story telling because such can affect the child's meaning making as they grow and develop.

Primary school aged children – the risk at this time of development is that the child can attribute the death of a significant other to their own magical thinking (the belief that their thoughts can influence events). Many observations of school aged children are equivocal to those seen in pre-schoolers. The gradual exposure to loss through childhood through being told or reading fairy tales, through the loss of older family members and pets can increase their awareness and understanding of death and can assist with their coping abilities.

Adolescence – This developmental stage spans 12–19 years. However, there is some debate that identity formation continues into our late twenties. Neuroscientists confer that the reintegration of the prefrontal cortex is complete by age 25 (Siegel, 2020). Erikson's theory of development is relevant in understanding the child's diffusion of identity as the period of adolescence tasks itself with the child finding stable ground to differentiate from their families. This period of rapid growth and changing self-perceptions can intensify reaction to death and other losses. Christ et al. (2002) state that children in early adolescence remain ego centric where older adolescents can respect that others are grieving too. Until adolescence children spend more time not thinking about grief. In adolescence the time spent thinking and not thinking about grief is let predictable as they transition to adulthood where adults in comparison spend more time than children thinking about the grief/mourning. Adolescents are faced with a double jeopardy in that they try to be not too over emotional because they perceive it to be childish or are trying to be less expressive to fit with a more adult role (Kentor and Kaplow, 2020). Interventions that allow grief processing whilst doing other activities are most beneficial. For example, those that involve creativity (song writing, crafting, dance), these are more acceptable than play or direct talking therapies. Wilkinson et al. (2013) identify that the more introverted teens are more prone to depression and so interventions that promote distraction are especially supportive for them.

Young adults – With delayed entry into the workplace and financial dependence continued with parents to a later age than historically, young adulthood is being delayed into the mid-twenties (Furstenberg et al., 2004). Stein et al. (2009) state that the death of a loved one can also hinder or moderate young adult's development. Where a death is anticipated it is typically less distressing. Bereaved young adults will aim to continue life as usual, regardless of their suffering, to show everyone and themselves that they can get through life OK alone. Neimeyer et al. (2006) found that in exploring continuing bonds with meaning making helped young adults to experience fewer symptoms of complicated grief, indeed some were also able to see transformational positives in their loss. Enabling young adults to tell their story allows them to adjust better.

Middle adulthood – with the extended years of young adulthood, middle adulthood can be extended to 50–70 years of age. Once we reach middle age, we become reflective of our lives lived so far. With a heightened sense of our own mortality, we begin to think about generativity – making life contributions that will be meaningful to significant others and even on a wider scale that will transcend our deaths. Losing a child at this age can cloud all judgments. The obsession with generativity increases the effect because the child and their children or future children were to benefit from the production and reception of their generativity. This can induce two responses of feeling, one of life now being meaningless to one where there is a feeling of heightened meaningfulness because the temporality of life has been made more explicit.

Middle aged adults find themselves in receipt of much support not least because peers have more experience of loss at this age. It is important that middle aged adults are encouraged to maintain continued bonds with the deceased but to also maintain relations with the living, to help them express and find meaning in the loss and to embrace shifts in identity. It is at this age that bereavement groups can be viewed the most supportive, verbalising experiences with others is also welcomed (Wortman et al., 2008).

The nature of the bereavement

Both developmental psychologists and sociologists acknowledge the importance of social relationships in our developmental wellbeing. There are also studies that suggest the death of a family member can impact upon the bereaved person's physical health. There are differences observed however in terms of the nature of the relationship and the biopsychosocial responses that follow.

Losing a parent in childhood

Bereavement is one of many events that can happen in childhood and impact on the child's developmental wellbeing. The experience of the loss of a parent in childhood is not rare. Parsons (2011) suggests that once a child has reached sixteen years old, they have a 4.7% chance of having lost one or both parents. This equates to approximately one in twenty young people. The last UK survey to establish prevalence of this type of loss was conducted in 2004. This data suggested that approximately 3.5% of 5–16-year-olds had lost a parent or a sibling, equating to one out of twenty-nine or on average one child per school classroom) (Costelloe et al., 2020). Looking at the total population of the UK, this suggests that approximately 309,000 school age children will have suffered this significant bereavement. Mortality rates are falling so it is likely that parental death rates could have also since reduced.

Meyer-Lee et al. (2020) explore the impacts of bereavement in childhood and indicate that affects can be both short and long term, especially with the loss of a parent (significantly more so if a child loses their mother). Effects include poor educational and employment achievements, leaving home early, early sexual and partnering activities, delinquency, depression and lowered or diminished self-concept and self-esteem.

Further, we should not neglect those young adults who are caring for loved ones who are dying. Romm (2009) in her memoir, openly describes her experience as she cares for her mother who is dying from cancer. She is supportive of her family through the disease process, but her own grief, upset and fears are evident:

> Romm (2009) May 17th the Guardian: *'And I realise now, in the dark room, that I am not ready, that I will never be ready, that her death will change me even though I've understood that it's been coming for nine years. And all the changes won't be hopeful – like the clarity of vision I sometimes feel when I'm in my bedroom after crying and the lines of the windows and slatted doors all look too sharp, hypersharp, and all people seem tragic and plain to me, easy to understand. Some of the changes will be only pain. Pain when I see babies, pain when my friends go to lunch with their mothers, pain on my birthday, on her birthday, on every birthday of every person I know. Pain and a deep, toothy hollowness inside me that will go on grinding forever'.*

Sibling loss

The relationships we hold with our siblings are unique. Siblings are there to learn from each other and to support each other, with bonds different to any other relationship we will encounter (Jensen et al., 2018). When siblings are gravely ill, the impact can therefore be profound, altering familial and personal identities and the confidence the healthy sibling may have in navigating their worlds (Wilkins and Woodgate, 2007). When a sibling dies, the living sibling also often loses their friend and role model (Davies, 2016).

There is limited research that has explored sibling relationships and perspectives throughout serious illness and death. The studies are more concentrated upon the impact of the bereavement rather than the anticipatory grief which itself can have influence on bereavement outcomes. In studies three to twelve months post death, siblings have been found to be socially withdrawn with low levels of social competence as compared to none bereaved matched age samples. These social characteristics can also be linked to later in life social difficulties (Foster et al., 2012). Barrera et al. (2013) suggest that bereaved siblings in childhood can manifest psychological difficulties, showing amongst them higher levels of anxiety and depression, low self-esteem and for younger children real difficulty in grasping the permanence of death and the fact that their sibling is not to return and share their day to day lives with them.

There are, however, always exceptions and some siblings have been found to psychosocially advance following the death of their sibling, showing increased maturity, self-esteem and compassion for others (Eilegard et al., 2013; Foster et al., 2012). A contemporary longitudinal study conducted by Eaton Russell et al. (2018) recruited 10 siblings, following them whilst living with a gravely ill child for two years. The study offers important insights to the worlds of young people going through this experience. Each reported incidences of strength and strain. They welcomed being involved with the cares of the sick child and to be involved in the anticipatory grief that transitions in the child's condition brought for their parents and families. The family time was deemed precious and helped their perceived resilience but the respondents of the participants of the study were often mindful that this time cost them time with peers and often the demands of the child's illness and the related worry was the dictator of their day-to-day thoughts and overshadowed their activities.

The parental loss of a child

The loss of a child is deemed incomparable to any other loss with grief responses regarded as more intense, longer lasting and life altering. Bereaved parents are also more likely to have elevated levels of depressive and anxiety symptoms (Kreicbergs et al., 2004), with an increased risk of post-traumatic stress disorder and the need for mental health care (Ljungman et al., 2015). Bereaved parents can also have marital issues and poor health-related quality of life, increasing their risk of mortality within the first three years post death (Song et al., 2010). In addition, where children experience pain at the end of life, this can add to parental grief (Wolfe et al., 2000).

Social support is associated with more positive responses amongst parents. Where this is not available or not accessed there is a higher risk of more complicated grief (Villacieros et al., 2014). Good marital relationships also link to less complex grief responses (Song et al., 2010). Parents also value the support of professionals. Supportive relationships between health and social care professionals and the families of deceased children are important because parents perceive that they are the ones who can empathise mostly with their realities (Garstang et al., 2014). However, many studies identify that continued contact varies, if there is follow up it is often informally. As such, families would benefit if cares were continued through a period of a parent's bereavement formally, not least because hectic work schedules limit the time professionals can do such informally which can mean families are cut off from the support they deem most valuable.

The search for meaning for parents is paramount to their adjustment, maintaining the memory of the child is important. Klass (1997) suggested that parents adapt through a continued integration of their child in their lives, albeit in a different capacity. Trying to deny the strong bonds that exist between a parent and child, does not help families to cope.

The loss of a partner/spouse

Many studies over the years have explored the loss of a spouse, but most have focused on bereaved widows (Nolen Hoeksema et al., 1997). A spouse is defined as a married partner, however the research to date has also addressed the needs of none married partners. Losing a partner is rated one of the most stressful events in life. Levels of stress do decrease with time but are extremely high in the immediacy of the death (Bonanno et al., 2002). Because studies are more focused on female samples it is difficult to draw gender related conclusions. This type of bereavement puts survivors at increased risk of mental health difficulties and Manor and Eisenbach (2003) found an elevated risk of mortality in the initial couple of years post bereavement. Majid and Ennis (2022) also highlight how existent health conditions can be exacerbated following the death of a partner. The younger the bereaved the more vulnerable they are (Zisook and Schucter, 1991) as well as those individuals in the lower end of the social spectrum (Martikainen and Valkonen, 1998). Younger widows and widowers also exhibit increased psychopathy compared to those in the older age groups (Zisook and Schucter, 1991).

Bonanno et al. (2002) identified that the biggest predictor of complicated grief was overdependence in the relationship. The widow's ability to cognitively adapt and show positivity for their futures was identified by O'Rourke (2004) to positively influence life satisfaction and reduce psychological distress.

Spiritual and cultural aspects of bereavement

The nature of the bereavement impacts on the affect. Culture can dictate to what extent the emotionality of the affect can be played out socially. In some cultures, death and mourning is a communal event, for others it is more private and somber. There are no studies that have identified that one type of mourning is more beneficial than another, it is important then that in practice we are accepting of diverse cultures ways of doing things. When families have rituals and practices to hinge upon, they can help the grieving processes of the bereaved (Parkes, 1997; Doka, 2002).

Spiritual matters that are related to death are of cultural importance. Funerals and related rituals facilitate transitions regardless of the nature of the bereavement. They also provide the opportunity for a public display of grief. For many western cultures however, there is a lack of continued ritual or direction. This can be difficult for some people because there is no template of how one should behave. Being supported in this time and allowed to grieve can be of longer-term importance (Mitima-Verloop et al., 2021).

Meaning reconstruction following loss

Meaning making allows the bereaved to make sense out of their loss and to rebuild their world views. An individual's ability to make meaning out of the death of a loved one can be influenced by how the person died. When the loss is categorised or experienced as traumatic, people turn to philosophical and spiritual resources for comfort and understanding (Lichtenthal et al., 2013). An individual's ability to make sense of the loss seems to be more predictive of whether the grief will become complicated or whether it will take a more 'normative' course of adjusting and moving forward over time (Currier et al., 2006; Holland et al., 2006; Lichtenthal et al., 2013; Majid and Ennis, 2022). Developing an enhanced appreciation of life was something that Lichtenthal et al. (2013) discovered in researching parents who had suffered the violent loss of their child, that the death increased their understanding and perception that life is precious and fleeting. Violent death often leads to a greater appreciation of relationships and researchers have found death by suicide leads parents to re-evaluate their lives and strive for purpose going forward (Lichtenthal et al., 2013). Following traumatic loss, if the bereaved are able to frame the loss as gods will or that the spirit will live on or that one day they may be reunited and if they believe that it is life and so bad things happen, then they are more able to perceive death as holding some meaning in the scheme of life.

An individual's ability to make sense of the loss also appears predictive of whether the grief will materialize as complicated or not. However, there is a body of research that suggests finding meaning can be difficult. Making sense of a loss is not an easy task and many bereaved individuals can be overburdened with the loss they are experiencing. So much so that they cannot accommodate the fact as reality. In parents this denial can lead to longer term mental health difficulties and the failure to link to a religious or spiritual meaning can further complicate their grief.

Most definitions of meaning making in the context of loss and bereavement involve two distinct processes:

1. Making sense of the loss (e.g., the death was in some manner inevitable; it is congruent with the caregiver's belief system which itself can provide some level of meaning); and
2. Finding benefits from the loss (e.g., it developed a strength of character and of identity and relationships with other significant others).

Finding benefits from the loss can be related to the concept of post-traumatic growth (Davis, 2008). The associated literature is focused on the positive changes that can occur in those bereaved and because of the loss. For example, the experience can mean individuals develop a more intense self-awareness, appreciation of relationships or reorder their own life priorities in the view that their lives will hold more purpose. Individuals make meaning out of a loss also with respect to their core beliefs around issues of fairness, benevolence, and predictability (Stein et al., 2018).

Other authors view this type of personal growth as a coping strategy. Davis (2008) reviewed a number of meaning making models and the post traumatic growth literature and suggested that some coping styles involve a change in attitude and in values but not longer-term changes. These however can be seen to be brought about by the post traumatic growth. Studies of grief and attachment (Field and Filanosky, 2010; Scholtes and Browne, 2015) highlight positive correlations between scores on some subscales of continuing bonds and scores on posttraumatic growth measures (Field and Filanosky, 2010). A greater understanding of continuing bonds and of post-traumatic growth is needed to understand how the bereaved make meaning of their losses. Such research with children and young people, particularly siblings would possibly enable psychological strategies or interventions for families to support their coping through anticipatory grief and bereavement.

Complications of bereavement

Just over a century ago, Freud (1917/1957) wrote:

> *Although mourning involves grave departures from the normal attitude toward life, it never occurs to us to regard it as a pathological condition and to refer it to a medical treatment. We rely on its being overcome after a certain lapse of time, and we look upon any interference with it as useless or even harmful.*
>
> (p. 243)

Studies since have in some ways supported Freud's conceptualisation. The pain of grief for a minority of the bereaved can be so strong and long lasting. At risk individuals are those whose bereavements have been unexpected, traumatic or against life's natural order of events, in the instance of losing a child. Complicated grief (CG) or more recently termed prolonged grief disorder (PGD), has received much attention in recent years by both psychiatrists and psychologists. Acute grief is a normal response to loss, however when the intensity continues for extended periods of time and there are difficulties for the person to maintain any level of equilibrium, then there may be a need for intervention.

Prolonged grief disorder and the DSM-V

It is estimated that between 10 to 20% of those bereaved have complicated or prolonged grief (Bonanno et al., 2002). More recent studies use the term

'Prolonged Grief Disorder' (PGD) (Jordan and Litz, 2014). PGD is often present alongside other mental health difficulties such as depression and PTSD, but it can be a distinct condition. Those with PGD can experience both physical and psychological symptoms that include increased thoughts of suicide, increased risk of heart problems, substance use and sleep difficulties. Other symptoms can include:

1. Chronic separation distress (a great longing for the deceased, loneliness, and a mind that is overwhelmed by thoughts of the deceased).
2. Symptoms of traumatic distress (feelings of disbelief, mistrust, anger, shock, detachment from others, and experiencing somatic symptoms of the deceased) (Lobb et al., 2010).

Although death is a natural phenomenon, and most people will independently adapt. Others can have more problems in meaning making, struggling to reframe relationships and the memories of the deceased into their continued lives. Where struggles continue there is also the risk of developing PTSD (Dyregrov et al., 2015).

> *PTSD is characterized typically by fear, horror, anger, guilt, or shame, combined with an anxious hyperarousal and exaggerated reactivity, the experience of PGD is marked primarily by yearning, loss, or emptiness.*
>
> (Jordan and Litz, 2014, p. 182)

Those with PGD can also have intrusive thoughts of the deceased (Jordan and Litz, 2014).

The inclusion of complicated grief in the DSM-V has received a lot of support. Not least because those suffering, experience difficulties that many will brush off as normal grief and this leaves the affected lost with no instrumental help. If their struggle is recognised and even if that means giving the struggle a medical label, it means that they hopefully can access professional support to be able to return to a normal sense of self and cope with everyday demands of life. Applying such labels globally however needs to be done so with caution (Rosenblatt, 2013).

Cultural contexts always need to be considered. Hsu et al. (2002) state that Taiwanese widows do not cry in front of the body of the deceased but after the funeral they can cry as much as they like. Alternatively, African Americans are encouraged to show intense public grieving. A further example is the norms for maternal grieving in Egypt. A period of intense grieving of up to seven years would not be considered as complex or as a PGD. The bereaved Balinese are also expected to grieve intensely and if they do not then they are behaving inappropriately. In some African cultures it is also perceived as normal to believe the bereaved are possessed by the spirits of the dead. As such, we can only make diagnostic conclusions about complicated grief if we also account for cultural norms and differences (Rosenblatt and Wallace, 2005; Wikan, 1988).

Further factors influencing bereavement outcome

Characteristics of the bereaved

Personality traits can impact on how we deal with loss. Trait anxiety, depression, neuroticism, satisfaction with life and being emotionally fragile are each related to emotional burden (Ferrario et al., 2004). Females in general also report greater psychological distress in bereavement than males. Age is also a predictor of distress although results are conflicting. Some studies suggest older carers have more complex grief reactions. In contract, caregivers of younger individuals have been found to have higher levels of depression (Ferrario et al., 2004). Experience of childhood parental separation, previous familial bereavement and individual coping styles are all looked upon as predictive variables of levels of bereavement distress (Boelen and Lenferink, 2020).

Care-giving experience

Care-giving impacts on emotional and physical wellbeing and can affect social integration and employment opportunities. Caregivers who report limited social support and a decline in their physical health experience poorer mental health post bereavement. In contrast, decreasing the caregiver burden can result in lower levels of bereavement distress (Delalibera et al., 2020).

Social support and family functioning

Low levels of social support relate to short term bereavement distress (Cohen and McKay, 2020). It is unclear however, what type and frequency of support is available for those bereaved. For example, The Childhood Bereavement Network conducted a survey of all local authorities and Primary Care Trusts in England in 2009. They were unable to determine the nature of any accessible support (Penny, 2010). The low response rate of 35% also could suggest the level of importance placed on such provision in mainstream services. However, current policy does now offer more support for these types of services, especially in areas deemed to be disadvantaged (Rolls, 2019). In the questionnaires returned in the survey, most responses suggested that bereaved children's needs were addressed through general care plans and related strategies and if needed via Child and Adolescent Mental Health Services (CAMHS) (Penny, 2010). A repeat survey would be of interest, to explore the availability of current provision, uptake and impact.

Preparation for and place of death

The place of death can be an important consideration for the 'good death' from the perspective of individuals and families. In addition, a lack of preparation for such can be a risk factor for later distress and psychological difficulties. Where the bereaved have the support of friends and family they can be more prepared for death and then more able to adapt to their bereavement.

Death at home is linked with lower levels of distress in initial bereavement but compared to other bereaved individuals at six months, there are no significant differences reported. When the death happens at home however, the happening is associated with a better general mental health of the caregiver. Although there are studies that have noted higher levels of distress for relatives when death occurs at home. This maybe because of the related care giver burden on the nature of the death itself (Morris et al., 2015).

When children die in the hospital setting, parents struggle with higher levels of psychological distress, depression, and paternal anxiety. Professionals increasingly promote choice in place of death, and this is something that should be revisited regularly with parents/families as the reality of the dying becomes closer in sight (Morris et al., 2019).

Chapter summary

Loss and grief are an intrinsic part of our human existence. Grief is an all-encompassing emotional and embodied experience that can manifest in psychological difficulties for some. However, most manifestations are time bound or the loss can become increasingly managed so that the bereaved can reconceptualise their life and being and begin to accommodate such in their lives left to live. Grief is the result of relationships, of emotional bonds made with others and loss itself and the disconnectedness it creates can be difficult to manage.

The literature around grief and bereavement has evolved over the years to appreciate that how one may experience any loss cannot be predicated and the experience itself cannot always be compartmentalised into any stage or pattern of behavioural response. There is a lack of support for example for grief being a predictable emotional trajectory, grieving moves the bereaved from a place of distress to a place 'recovery'. We are also no longer working with the belief that to successfully adapt to a loss or to manage the bereavement then there must be a 'letting go' of the deceased. Instead, we recognise that maintaining a continued bond with the diseased can be emotionally helpful.

Mainstream research has contoured our understanding of grief and bereavement and expressions of such involves risk factors, distinct symptoms, and psychological processes, but the one size fits all notion cannot be justified. Support must be mindful of the unique characteristics of the sufferer, the psychological wellbeing before the death, how the significant other died, what the relationship to the deceased was, what culture they belong to and what support networks are available to them.

To both understand grief and to accommodate it we need to accept that the experience is nuanced, it is private and social and so we need to embrace broader perspectives in our psychological interpretations of 'normal' or 'complex'.

Key issues

1. Dominant medical discourse on grief and bereavement was historically dictated by Freud's original theorisation of grief and grief work, which contended that to 'recover' there needed to be a detachment from the deceased.
2. Since Freud's theoretical conception there has been a multitude of grief theories proposed. Many have continued to use the discourse of 'moving on' and 'letting go' via time bound or stage models. These theories promote an adjusting to life without the deceased, further categorising normal and abnormal grief pathways. The work of Bowlby and Parkes redefined the work of Kubler Ross, influencing the work of palliative care and hospice provision. As such, we to continue to be mindful of the value of attachment theory and in understanding the normative behavioural responses associated with separation anxiety that can occur through facing and living with grief and bereavement.
3. Current understandings of grief and bereavement are multifaceted, and are considerate of personal and social variables. Grief itself, however, is relational.
4. Where there is complex grief, where the bereavement is off time or traumatic, continuing bonds can particularly assist meaning making.

Box 8.1 Reflective questions

1. Have you been bereaved? (Was the experience relational? Time bound?)
2. Does the experience of bereavement change worldviews?

References

Attig, T., 2012. Reaching through sorrow to legacy. *Techniques of Grief Therapy: Creative Practices for Counseling the Bereaved* (pp. 277–280). Routledge.

Barrera, M., Alam, R., D'Agostino, N.M., Nicholas, D.B. and Schneiderman, G., 2013. Parental perceptions of siblings' grieving after a childhood cancer death: A longitudinal study. *Death Studies*, *37*(1), pp.25–46.

Boelen, P.A. and Lenferink, L.I., 2020. Symptoms of prolonged grief, posttraumatic stress, and depression in recently bereaved people: Symptom profiles, predictive value, and cognitive behavioural correlates. *Social Psychiatry and Psychiatric Epidemiology*, *55*(6), pp.765–777.

Boerner, K. and Heckhausen, J., 2003. To have and have not: Adaptive bereavement by transforming mental ties to the deceased. *Death Studies*, *27*(3), pp.199–226.

Bonanno, G.A., Papa, A., Lalande, K., Westphal, M. and Coifman, K., 2004. The importance of being flexible: The ability to both enhance and suppress emotional expression predicts long-term adjustment. *Psychological Science, 15*(7), pp.482–487.

Bonanno, G.A., Wortman, C.B., Lehman, D.R., Tweed, R.G., Haring, M., Sonnega, J., Carr, D. and Nesse, R.M., 2002. Resilience to loss and chronic grief: A prospective study from preloss to 18-months postloss. *Journal of Personality and Social Psychology, 83*(5), p.1150.

Bowlby, J., 1980. Attachment and loss: Volume III: Loss, sadness and depression. In *Attachment and Loss: Volume III: Loss, Sadness and Depression* (pp. 1–462). The Hogarth Press and the Institute of Psychoanalysis.

Christ, G.H., Siegel, K. and Christ, A.E., 2002. Adolescent grief: It never really hit me... until it actually happened. *Jama, 288*(10), pp.1269–1278.

Coates, S. and Gaensbauer, T.J., 2009. Event trauma in early childhood: symptoms, assessment, intervention. *Child and Adolescent Psychiatric Clinics, 18*(3), pp.611–626.

Cohen, S. and McKay, G., 2020. Social support, stress and the buffering hypothesis: A theoretical analysis. In *Handbook of Psychology and Health (Volume IV)* (pp. 253–267). Routledge.

Costelloe, A., Mintz, J. and Lee, F., 2020. Bereavement support provision in primary schools: an exploratory study. *Educational Psychology in Practice, 36*(3), pp.281–296.

Currier, J.M., Holland, J.M. and Neimeyer, R.A., 2006. Sense-making, grief, and the experience of violent loss: Toward a mediational model. *Death Studies, 30*(5), pp.403–428.

Currier, J.M., Holland, J.M. and Neimeyer, R.A., 2007. The effectiveness of bereavement interventions with children: A meta-analytic review of controlled outcome research. *Journal of Clinical Child and Adolescent Psychology, 36*(2), pp.253–259.

Datson Samuel, J. and Marwit, S., 1997. Personality constructs and perceived presence of deceased loved ones. *Death Studies, 21*(2), pp.131–146.

Davies, B., 2016. Shadows in the sun: Towards understanding the grief of young siblings. In *Sibling Loss Across the Lifespan* (pp. 49–56). Routledge.

Davis, C.G., 2008. Redefining goals and redefining self: A closer look at posttraumatic growth following loss.

Delalibera, M., Coelho, A., Frade, P., Barbosa, A. and Leal, I., 2020. Caregiving and bereavement in palliative care: A cross-cultural study between Brazil and Portugal. *Transcultural Psychiatry, 57*(3), pp.445–454.

Doka, K., 2002. How could God. In J. Kauffman (Ed.), *Loss of the Assumptive World: A Theory of Traumatic Loss* (pp.49–54). Routledge.

Doka, K.J., 2008. Disenfranchised grief in historical and cultural perspective. In M. S. Stroebe, R. O. Hansson, H. Schut and W. Stroebe (Eds.), *Handbook of Bereavement Research: Consequences, Coping, and Care* (pp. 223–240). American Psychological Association.

Dyregrov, A., Salloum, A., Kristensen, P. and Dyregrov, K., 2015. Grief and traumatic grief in children in the context of mass trauma. *Current Psychiatry Reports, 17*(6), pp.1–8.

Eaton Russell, C., Widger, K., Beaune, L., Neville, A., Cadell, S., Steele, R., Rapoport, A., Rugg, M. and Barrera, M., 2018. Siblings' voices: A prospective investigation of experiences with a dying child. *Death Studies, 42*(3), pp.184–194.

Eilegård, A., Steineck, G., Nyberg, T. and Kreicbergs, U., 2013. Psychological health in siblings who lost a brother or sister to cancer 2 to 9 years earlier. *Psycho-Oncology, 22*(3), pp.683–691.

Ferrario, S.R., Cardillo, V., Vicario, F., Balzarini, E. and Zotti, A.M., 2004. Advanced cancer at home: caregiving and bereavement. *Palliative Medicine*, *18*(2), pp.129–136.

Field, N.P. and Filanosky, C., 2009. Continuing bonds, risk factors for complicated grief, and adjustment to bereavement. *Death Studies*, *34*(1), pp.1–29.

Field, N.P. and Filanosky, C., 2010. Continuing bonds, risk factors for complicated grief, and adjustment to bereavement. *Death Studies*, *34*(1), pp.1–29.

Field, N.P., 2006. Continuing bonds in adaptation to bereavement: Introduction. *Death Studies*, *30*(8), pp.709–714.

Field, T.F., Choppa, A.J., Johnson, C.B., Jayne, K.A., Fountaine, J.D. and Smith, A.M., 2008. Bereavement and mortality: a methodology for assessing capacity and functioning following the loss of a spouse. *Journal of Life Care Planning*, 7(4), pp.163–179.

Foster, T.L., Gilmer, M.J., Vannatta, K., Barrera, M., Davies, B., Dietrich, M.S., Fairclough, D.L. and Gerhardt, C.A., 2012. Changes in siblings after the death of a child from cancer. *Cancer Nursing*, *35*(5), p.347.

Freud, S., 1917/1957. Mourning and melancholia. *Standard Edition*, *14*(239), pp.1957–1961.

Friedman, R. and James, J.W., 2008. The myth of the stages of dying, death and grief. *Skeptic* (Altadena, CA), *14*(2), pp.37–42.

Furstenberg Jr, F.F., Kennedy, S., McLoyd, V.C., Rumbaut, R.G. and Settersten Jr, R.A., 2004. Growing up is harder to do. *Contexts*, *3*(3), pp.33–41.

Garstang, J., Griffiths, F. and Sidebotham, P., 2014. What do bereaved parents want from professionals after the sudden death of their child: A systematic review of the literature. *BMC Pediatrics*, *14*(1), pp.1–17.

Gerhardt, C.A., Fairclough, D.L., Grossenbacher, J.C., Barrera, M., Jo Gilmer, M., Foster, T.L., Compas, B.E., Davies, B., Hogan, N.S. and Vannatta, K., 2012. Peer relationships of bereaved siblings and comparison classmates after a child's death from cancer. *Journal of Pediatric Psychology*, *37*(2), pp.209–219.

Hale, G., 1996. The social construction of grief. *Integrating Perspectives On Health*, p.110.

Holland, J.M., Currier, J.M. and Neimeyer, R.A., 2006. Meaning reconstruction in the first two years of bereavement: The role of sense-making and benefit-finding. *Omega-Journal of Death and Dying*, *53*(3), pp.175–191.

Hsu, M.T., Kahn, D.L. and Hsu, M., 2002. A single leaf orchid: Meaning of a husband's death for Taiwanese widows. *Ethos*, *30*(4), pp.306–326.

Hsu, M.T., Kahn, D.L., Yee, D.H. and Lee, W.L., 2004. Recovery through reconnection: A cultural design for family bereavement in Taiwan. *Death Studies*, *28*(8), pp.761–786.

Jensen, A.C., Whiteman, S.D. and Fingerman, K.L., 2018. 'Can't live with or without them:' Transitions and young adults' perceptions of sibling relationships. *Journal of Family Psychology*, *32*(3), p.385.

Jordan, A.H. and Litz, B.T., 2014. Prolonged grief disorder: diagnostic, assessment, and treatment considerations. *Professional Psychology: Research and Practice*, *45*(3), p.180.

Kauffman, J. ed., 2011. *The Shame Of Death, Grief, and Trauma*. Routledge.

Kentor, R.A. and Kaplow, J.B., 2020. Supporting children and adolescents following parental bereavement: guidance for health-care professionals. *The Lancet Child & Adolescent Health*, *4*(12), pp.889–898.

Kessler, D., 2004. The extraordinary ordinary death of Elisabeth Kübler-Ross. *American Journal of Hospice and Palliative Medicine*, *21*(6), 415–416.

Klass, D. and Walter, T., 2001. Processes of grieving: How bonds are continued. In M. S. Stroebe, R. O. Hansson, W. Stroebe, and H. Schut (Eds.), *Handbook of Bereavement*

Research: Consequences, Coping, and Care (pp. 431–448). American Psychological Association.

Klass, D., 1993. Solace and immortality: Bereaved parents' continuing bond with their children. *Death Studies*, *17*(4), pp.343–368.

Klass, D., 1997. The deceased child in the psychic and social worlds of bereaved parents during the resolution of grief. *Death Studies*, *21*(2), pp.147–176.

Klass, D., 2006. Continuing conversation about continuing bonds. *Death Studies*, *30*(9), pp.843–858.

Kreicbergs, U., Valdimarsdóttir, U., Onelöv, E., Henter, J.I. and Steineck, G., 2004. Talking about death with children who have severe malignant disease. *New England Journal of Medicine*, *351*(12), pp.1175–1186.

Kübler-Ross, E. and Kessler, D., 2005. *On Grief and Grieving: Finding the Meaning of Grief Through the Five Stages of Loss*. Simon and Schuster.

Kübler-Ross, E., 1969. *On Death and Dying*. Macmillan.

Li, J., Stroebe, M., Chan, C.L. and Chow, A.Y., 2014. Guilt in bereavement: A review and conceptual framework. *Death Studies*, *38*(3), pp.165–171.

Lichtenthal, W.G., Neimeyer, R.A., Currier, J.M., Roberts, K. and Jordan, N., 2013. Cause of death and the quest for meaning after the loss of a child. *Death Studies*, *37*(4), pp.311–342.

Ljungman, L., Hovén, E., Ljungman, G., Cernvall, M. and von Essen, L., 2015. Does time heal all wounds? A longitudinal study of the development of posttraumatic stress symptoms in parents of survivors of childhood cancer and bereaved parents. *Psycho-Oncology*, *24*(12), pp.1792–1798.

Lobb, E.A., Kristjanson, L.J., Aoun, S.M., Monterosso, L., Halkett, G.K. and Davies, A., 2010. Predictors of complicated grief: A systematic review of empirical studies. *Death Studies*, *34*(8), pp.673–698.

Majid, U. and Ennis, J., 2022. "Continuing the cConnection" or "Carrying On"? A qualitative evidence synthesis of how widows explain the physical health outcomes after spousal loss. *The Family Journal*, *30*(1), pp.111–118.

Manor, O. and Eisenbach, Z., 2003. Mortality after spousal loss: are there socio-demographic differences? *Social Science & Medicine*, *56*(2), pp.405–413.

Markese, S., 2013. Dyadic trauma in infancy and early childhood: Review of the literature. *Mothers, Infants and Young Children of September 11, 2001*, pp.206–243.

Martikainen, P. and Valkonen, T., 1998. Do education and income buffer the effects of death of spouse on mortality? *Epidemiology*, pp.530–534.

Meyer-Lee, C.B., Jackson, J.B. and Gutierrez, N.S., 2020. Long-term experiencing of parental death during childhood: a qualitative analysis. *The Family Journal*, *28*(3), pp.247–256.

Mitima-Verloop, H.B., Mooren, T.T. and Boelen, P.A., 2021. Facilitating grief: An exploration of the function of funerals and rituals in relation to grief reactions. *Death Studies*, *45*(9), pp.735–745.

Morris, S., Fletcher, K. and Goldstein, R., 2019. The grief of parents after the death of a young child. *Journal of Clinical Psychology in Medical Settings*, *26*(3), pp.321–338.

Morris, S.M., King, C., Turner, M. and Payne, S., 2015. Family carers providing support to a person dying in the home setting: a narrative literature review. *Palliative Medicine*, *29*(6), pp.487–495.

Neimeyer, R.A. and Mahoney, M.J., 1996. Different paths to the same goal: The construction of constructivism in psychotherapy: Constructivism in psychotherapy. *Journal of Constructivist Psychology*, *9*(3), pp.233–247.

Neimeyer, R.A., 1998. Death anxiety research: The state of the art. *OMEGA-Journal of Death and Dying, 36*(2), pp.97–120.

Neimeyer, R.A., Baldwin, S.A. and Gillies, J., 2006. Continuing bonds and reconstructing meaning: Mitigating complications in bereavement. *Death Studies, 30*(8), pp.715–738.

Nolen-Hoeksema, S., McBride, A. and Larson, J., 1997. Rumination and psychological distress among bereaved partners. *Journal of Personality and Social Psychology, 72*(4), p.855.

O'Rourke, N., 2004. Psychological resilience and the well-being of widowed women. *Ageing International, 29*(3), pp.267–280.

Parkes, C.M., 1997. Bereavement and mental health in the elderly. *Reviews in Clinical Gerontology*, 7(1), pp.47–53.

Parkes, C.M., 1998. Traditional models and theories of grief. *Bereavement Care, 17*(2), pp.21–23.

Parsons, S., 2011. Long-term impact of childhood bereavement. *Preliminary Analysis of the 1970 British Cohort Study (BCS70).* Childhood Wellbeing Research Centre.

Penny, A., 2010. Childhood bereavement: the context and need for services. In B. Monroe and F. Kraus (Eds.), *Brief Interventions With Bereaved Children*, p.1–13, Oxford University Press.

Robson, P. and Walter, T., 2013. Hierarchies of loss: A critique of disenfranchised grief. *OMEGA-Journal of Death and Dying, 66*(2), pp.97–119.

Romm (2009) May 17th the Guardian: 'I know it's selfish, mum, but I can't tell you it's ok to die. I can't imagine life without you' www.theguardian.com/lifeandstyle/2009/may/17/robin-romm-mercy-papers-extract (accessed 15 May 2022).

Root, B.L. and Exline, J.J., 2014. The role of continuing bonds in coping with grief: Overview and future directions. *Death Studies, 38*(1), pp.1–8.

Rosenblatt, P.C. and Wallace, B.R., 2005. Narratives of grieving African Americans about racism in the lives of deceased family members. *Death Studies, 29*(3), pp.217–235.

Rosenblatt, P.C., 2008. Grief across cultures: A review and research agenda. In M. S. Stroebe, R. O. Hansson, H. Schut and W. Stroebe (Eds.), *Handbook of Bereavement Research: Consequences, Coping, and Care* (pp. 207–222). American Psychological Association.

Rosenblatt, P.C., 2013. *The Concept of Complicated Grief.* Scientific Foundations for Health Care Professionals.

Russac, R.J., Steighner, N.S. and Canto, A.I., 2002. Grief work versus continuing bonds: A call for paradigm integration or replacement? *Death Studies, 26*(6), pp.463–478.

Scholtes, D. and Browne, M., 2015. Internalized and externalized continuing bonds in bereaved parents: Their relationship with grief intensity and personal growth. *Death Studies, 39*(2), pp.75–83.

Shapiro, E.R., 2001. Grief in interpersonal perspective: Theories and their implications. In M. S. Stroebe, R. O. Hansson, W. Stroebe, and H. Schut (Eds.), *Handbook of Bereavement Research: Consequences, Coping, and Care* (pp. 301–327). American Psychological Association.

Siegel, D.J., 2020. *The developing Mind: How Relationships and the Brain Interact to Shape Who We Are.* Guilford Publications.

Song, J., Floyd, F.J., Seltzer, M.M., Greenberg, J.S. and Hong, J., 2010. Long-term effects of child death on parents' health-related quality of life: A dyadic analysis. *Family Relations, 59*(3), pp.269–282.

Stein, J.Y., Levin, Y., Bachem, R. and Solomon, Z., 2018. Growing apart: A longitudinal assessment of the relation between post-traumatic growth and loneliness among combat veterans. *Frontiers in Psychology*, *9*, p.893.

Stein, M.K., Smith, M.S., Henningsen, M.A. and Silver, E.A., 2009. *Implementing Standards-Based Math Instruction: A Casebook for Professional Development*. Teachers College Press.

Stroebe, M. and Schut, H., 2005. To continue or relinquish bonds: A review of consequences for the bereaved. *Death Studies*, *29*(6), pp.477–494.

Stroebe, M. and Schut, H., 2010. The dual process model of coping with bereavement: A decade on. *OMEGA-Journal of Death and Dying*, *61*(4), pp.273–289.

Stroebe, M. S., and Schut, H. (1999). The Dual Process Model of coping with bereavement: Rationale and description. *Death Studies*, *23*, pp. 197–224.

Stroebe, M., Schut, H. and Boerner, K., 2010. Continuing bonds in adaptation to bereavement: Toward theoretical integration. *Clinical* psychology review, *30*(2), pp.259–268.

Stroebe, M.S. and Archer, J., 2013. Origins of modern ideas on love and loss: Contrasting forerunners of attachment theory. *Review of General Psychology*, *17*(1), pp.28–39.

Valentine, C., 2006. Academic constructions of bereavement. *Mortality*, *11*(1), pp.57–78.

Villacieros, M., Serrano, I., Bermejo, J.C., Magaña, M. and Carabias, R., 2014. Social support and psychological well-being as possible predictors of complicated grief in a cross-section of people in mourning. [Apoyo social y bienestar psicológico como posibles predictores de estado de duelo complicado en poblac de personas en duelo]. *Anales de Psicología/Annals of Psychology*, *30*(3), pp.944–951.

Waugh, A., Kiemle, G. and Slade, P., 2018. What aspects of post-traumatic growth are experienced by bereaved parents? A systematic review. *European Journal of Psychotraumatology*, *9*(1), p.1506230.

Wikan, U., 1988. Bereavement and loss in two Muslim communities: Egypt and Bali compared. *Social Science & Medicine*, *27*(5), pp.451–460.

Wilkins, K.L. and Woodgate, R.L., 2007, March. An interruption in family life: siblings' lived experience as they transition through the pediatric bone marrow transplant trajectory. *Oncology Nursing Forum*, *34*(2), pp.E28–E35.

Wilkinson, P.O., Croudace, T.J. and Goodyer, I.M., 2013. Rumination, anxiety, depressive symptoms and subsequent depression in adolescents at risk for psychopathology: a longitudinal cohort study. *BMC Psychiatry*, *13*(1), pp.1–9.

Wolfe, J., Klar, N., Grier, H.E., Duncan, J., Salem-Schatz, S., Emanuel, E.J. and Weeks, J.C., 2000. Understanding of prognosis among parents of children who died of cancer: impact on treatment goals and integration of palliative care. *Jama*, *284*(19), pp.2469–2475.

Worden, J.W., 2018. *Grief Counseling and Grief Therapy: A Handbook for the Mental Health Practitioner*. Springer Publishing Company.

Wortmann, J.H. and Park, C.L., 2008. Religion and spirituality in adjustment following bereavement: An integrative review. *Death Studies*, *32*(8), pp.703–736.

Zisook, S. and Shuchter, S.R., 1991. Depression through the first year after the death of a spouse. *American Journal of Psychiatry*, *148*(10), pp.1346–1352.

Zisook, S., Simon, N.M., Reynolds III, C.F., Pies, R., Lebowitz, B., Young, I.T., Madowitz, J. and Shear, M.K., 2010. Bereavement, complicated grief, and DSM, part 2: complicated grief. *Journal of Clinical Psychiatry*, *71*(8), p.1869.

Epilogue

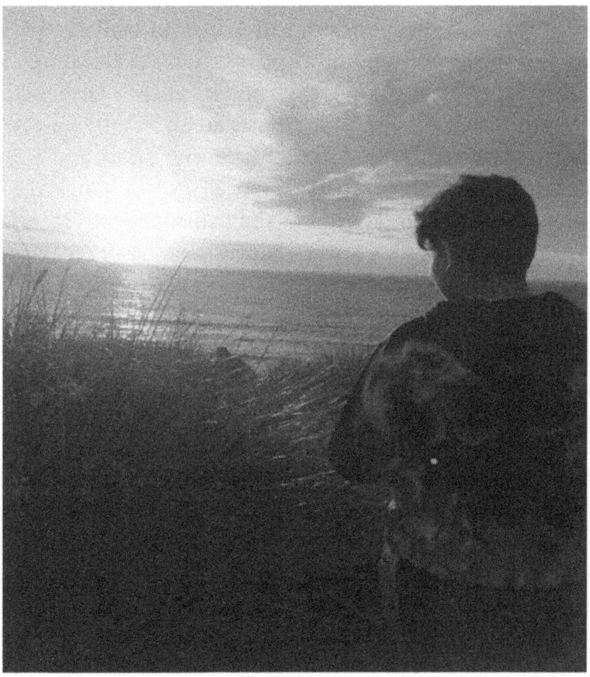

Epilogue Figure 1 A photograph of a young person looking out at the sun setting over the sea.

Photograph taken by Alison Rodriguez.

Death dying and palliative care: health psychology perspectives

Serious illness, death and dying for children and young people is a personal but familial experience supported in resource rich countries by formal palliative

DOI: 10.4324/9781003340287-10

care service provision. Delivered by generalist and specialist teams, palliative care provision for children and young people can be found in community and inpatient settings, continually evolving to meet the needs of the growing populations of individuals with life limiting/threatening conditions and their families. Existentialist philosophy identifies that we as human beings are universally characterised by our concern for meaning and purpose and this is heightened when we are faced with a serious illness and shortened life prognosis.

There is increasing awareness of children and young people's palliative care needs across areas of health and social care, hospice and in the community. The array of children and young people's palliative care services and guiding policy in the UK takes us from cradle through to transition to adulthood and for some into middle adulthood as they live longer with conditions that would have historically resulted in death in childhood. There are still however, areas of improvement to make, but in the last thirty years or so, our knowledge of death and dying experiences and the associated holistic care needs for children, young people and families in palliative care have grown significantly. The benefits of palliative care for children, young people and families are driven by an ethos of care which is individual and family centred. Empathy, compassion, and a mutuality of care are integral to good palliative care practice.

Medical intervention often remains central to the palliative care experience, with prognosis disclosure, illness information sharing and treatment barriers and needs receiving the most attention in the literature and being key elements of care processes. It has been beyond the scope of this book however, to begin to address mental health provision for children and young people with serious illness and their families, but we can note that there appears to be a void of specialist mental health support for individuals and families who are struggling through the experience of serious illness and advancing disease. This is also reflective of how health and social care provision has been impacted in general by austerity measures and has not been helped by the financial strain of the COVID-19 pandemic. Palliative care professionals however do seek to mitigate risks to mental health and aim to support families to support each other. Wellbeing may be further improved when and if communities can come together to share the care.

In the moment

Currently there is recognition that palliative care provided earlier in a disease trajectory can lead to better quality of life outcomes for children and young people with serious illness. We also have the tools to support effective symptom monitoring, information sharing, and care planning. There is a lot of motivation within the literature to meet the needs of individuals and family members at different developmental stages and with different mental capacities. However there remains the need to involve children and young people with serious illness more in studies so that we can understand their perspectives and needs better.

Health and social care professional education has developed to support undergraduate students in their quest to support the dying, with courses including education on palliative care measures and supportive processes. The EPICC movement (Enhancing Nurses' and Midwives' Competence in Providing Spiritual Care through Innovative Education and Compassionate Care) is also gathering pace to support the infiltration of spiritually compassionate care in undergraduate curriculums. With such actions, there is increased hope that the future nursing workforce will grow in empathic awareness of the needs of children and young people with serious illness and their families.

The last few years that have incorporated the COVID-19 pandemic have highlighted how communities can come together to celebrate life and to also mourn loss. The death positivity movement over recent years has promoted a more open attitude to death and dying, with active social media campaigns, death café interventions and festivals. These public events help in a small way to prepare us for what may come and to reduce the stigma and exclusion of individuals with serious illness and their families from societal participation. In addition, social media now allows us into the worlds of children and young people facing death and dying as they document and others report on their experiences. The fears that once were around social media are being replaced with an understanding that it is a means to promote social connectedness for children and young people with serious illness. Indeed, for children, young people and families, social media may be the only means they have to connect with peers at certain stages of disease trajectories, which is important for both psychological and developmental wellbeing. Loneliness can make the whole experience harder.

Looking out onto the horizon

There is more research to be done to explore how we can make young lives richer and care less burdensome for children, young people and families in receipt of palliative care. Extending the community reach of palliative care and finding ways for easier access to everyday activities for those with serious illnesses, could further positively influence shared attitudes and behaviours toward death, dying and palliative care. A more community integrated approach to care could lead to less social stigma for children and young people with serious illness, shifting attitudes away from viewing the seriously ill and disabled as more vulnerable with more need for protection than others. Key to perceptions of wellbeing for children and young people with serious illness is for their voices to be heard and valued and for them to be supported to live a life like others of their age and developmental stage – they strive to live a 'normal' life.

There exist complexities of communication within and between families, and sometimes these are resultant of the protectiveness triad that can occur between the child or young person, family and professional. The evidence base is recognising this and is proposing ways to help guide individuals to broach the more challenging conversations. In addition, there is a growing evidence base around the development of psycho-therapeutic interventions that incorporate activities to address psychological, spiritual, and existential concerns. Interventions such as life review and dignity therapy have proved to be beneficial for many individuals with serious illness and their families, providing a means for open conversations, sharing legacies and reducing death and dying related anxieties. There is much debate that continues around what constitutes a 'good death' or 'dying well'. Where individuals are supported to engage in psychotherapeutic interventions and can die with not having anything left to be said, there is the suggestion that they can have a sense of peace and mastery over their lives and reach a point of death acceptance.

Despite much creativity occurring in children's hospice settings that contribute to memory making, there is somewhat of a hesitance around developing formal psychosocial interventions that are for the purpose of memory making, life storying, meaning making and legacy leaving for children and young people. However, consultation work and research that has included the voices of children and young people is enabling the development of tailored psychotherapeutic approaches. These activities will encourage children and young people with serious illness to reflect on their lives and have an input into how they want to be remembered. This will help them and their families to appreciate that they have mattered, and that others will receive benefit from their memories and wisdom. There is psychological benefit for children and young people with serious illness who can understand that memories of them will have a positive influence on others. It is hoped that involvement in such projects will also be a means to have fun and enjoyment for them, enhancing their psychological wellbeing and coping more broadly.

Final note

Serious illness is an all-encompassing lived experience; the bodily impacts and care demands are felt psychologically, with individuals and families navigating their wellbeing by also drawing on social and spiritual resources. The anticipatory grief process that children, young people and their families encounter through their awareness of a shortened life expectancy and their experience of vulnerability impacts on their perceptions of care, relationships and emotions. This book has introduced readers to a range of topics, purposely selected to help them to begin to understand some of the more experiential health psychology perspectives relevant to children and young people living with serious illness and to understand some of the individual, practice and research needs within children's and young people's palliative care. It is hoped that readers can begin to develop an appreciation of the attitudes and behaviours that exist toward serious illness, death and dying in children and young people and that such will motivate their readiness to care, to share, to communicate and to facilitate support for this population – be that through their own practice, scholarship or research.

Index

For Product Safety Concerns and Information please contact our EU representative GPSR@taylorandfrancis.com
Taylor & Francis Verlag GmbH, Kaufingerstraße 24, 80331 München, Germany

www.ingramcontent.com/pod-product-compliance
Ingram Content Group UK Ltd.
Pitfield, Milton Keynes, MK11 3LW, UK
UKHW020140200926
475702UK00005B/836
* 9 7 8 1 0 3 2 3 7 4 4 0 6 *